Essential Oil Magic 2022

The Best Guide to Understanding the Natural Power of Essential Oil Magic

Copyright © 2022

No part of this publication may be reproduced, stored in a retrieval system, or transmitted in any form or by any means, electronic, mechanical, photocopying, recording, scanning, or otherwise, except as permitted under Sections 107 or 108 of the 1976 United States Copyright Act, without the prior written permission of the Publisher. Limit of Liability/Disclaimer of Warranty: The Publisher and the author make no representations or warranties with respect to the accuracy or completeness of the contents of this work and specifically disclaim all warranties, including without limitation warranties of fitness for a particular purpose. No warranty may be created or extended by sales or promotional materials. The advice and strategies contained herein may not be suitable for every situation. This work is sold with the understanding that the Publisher is not engaged in rendering medical, legal, or other professional advice or services. If professional assistance is required, the services of a competent professional person should be sought. Neither the Publisher nor the author shall be liable for damages arising herefrom. The fact that an individual, organization, or website is referred to in this work as a citation and/or potential source of further information does not mean that the author or the Publisher endorses the information the individual, organization, or website may provide or recommendations they/it may make. Further, readers should be aware that websites listed in this work may have changed or disappeared between when this work was written and when it is read.

CONTENTS

Introduction

PART I
Basics & Principles

CHAPTER 1
Principles of Magic

CHAPTER 2
The Magic of Essential Oils

PART II
Practical Magic

CHAPTER 3
On Essential Oils

CHAPTER 4
Working with Oils

CHAPTER 5
Practicing Magic

PART III
Magic Oils

CHAPTER 6

30 Magic Essential Oils

Basil

Black Pepper

Black Spruce

Cardamom

Cassia

Cedarwood

Chamomile

Citronella

Clary Sage

Clove

Eucalyptus

Frankincense

Geranium

Ginger

Helichrysum

Jasmine

Lavender

Lemon

Myrrh

Nutmeg

Orange

Patchouli

Peppermint

Rose
Rosemary
Sage
Sandalwood
Spearmint
Vetiver
Ylang Ylang

PART IV
Spells & Rituals

CHAPTER 7
Protection

Roll-On Energy Shield
Sacred Space Spray
Clear the Air
Protection Polish
Death's Own Cloak
No More Nightmares Pillow Spray
Front Door Defense
Four Corners Fortification
Auric Protection Pendant
Going Away Party

CHAPTER 8
Love

Self-Love Mirror Spell
Anahata Opening

Like a Moth to a Flame
Yummy Love Scrub
Goddess Body Wash
In the Mood for Love
Lovers' Massage Oil
Love Potion No. 10
Freyja's Necklace
Aphrodite's Bath

CHAPTER 9
Healing

Just Breathe
Soothing Salve
Inner Peace Inhaler
Moontime Roller
Wash Your Worries Away
Soothing Soak
Rest and Recover Roller
Summon the Sandman
Miracle Massage Oil
Happy Tummy Roller

CHAPTER 10
Wealth

Gratitude Journal
Abundance Mindset Inhaler
Pocket Pyrite
Make It Rain
Minting Money
Let the Good Times Roll

Liquid Gold Body Wash
Midas Touch Body Butter
Straw into Gold Hair Oil
Good Fortune Fizz

CHAPTER 11
Divination
Intuition Roller
Aura of Extrasensory Perception
Third Eye Anointing Oil
Divination Journal
Olfactory Oracle
Prophetic Dreams Pillow Spray
Get Intuit Anywhere
Inner Eye Illumination
Soothsayer's Soak
Rose Runes

Substitutions Chart
Glossary
Resources
References

INTRODUCTION

WELCOME TO THE world of oil magic! Perhaps you have stumbled into this world serendipitously, happening upon an oil or two (or maybe this book) and finding yourself curious about their magical potential. Or perhaps you have heard of oil magic before—and are curious to explore it for yourself. Maybe you are an expert in plant magic with fresh and dried herbs, and you've heard that essential oils possess the most potent plant magic of all. Maybe you even have some experience using essential oils for wellness and pleasure, but you are eager to expand your use of oils into the realm of magic. However you got here, I'm glad you came. Together, we will explore the use of essential oils in magic and spirituality—first historically, and then we'll look at the potential and methods for their use today.

Essential oils are extremely versatile magical allies. Through diffusion, essential oils can transform the energy of an environment. Worn as perfume, they can shift the energy of a person. Incorporated into personal care products and charms, they become powerful elements of simple but effective spells. As anointing oils, they can awaken and empower the subtle energy of crystals and other magical objects. Though they may not necessarily help you bottle fame or brew glory, they *can* help bewitch the mind and ensnare the senses. It would be too far a stretch to say they "put a stopper in death," but they *can* support the body in its natural healing process, through magic and other means.

I myself came to the oily side of the plant-magic path after years of exploring plant magic almost exclusively through tea (specifically the

Chinese art of *gong fu cha*) and cooking/kitchen witchery. I had heard of essential oils and purchased a few cheap oils here and there but didn't think much of them, and never used them for magic. When a critical mass of my friends had started using high-quality essential oils for their health and wellness, home and personal care, and spiritual practice, I saw firsthand how their lives were transformed and I wanted in. When I experienced their oils, I could tell that they were different. The cheap oils I had known could only be described as greenwashed home fragrance, whereas these *exuded positive qi.* I could feel the good vibes in my hand before even opening the bottles, and when I did open them, the aromas filled my senses (you could even say *ensnared* them) and shifted (or should I say *bewitched*?) my state of mind. I immediately sensed their magical potential and had to have them. So I purchased a set, studied and experimented, found recipes, and created my own. I made rollers, sprays, and diffuser blends for every intention imaginable, and my life began to change forever.

That experimentation and the research it inspired became the recipes, spells, potions, and miniature oil magic encyclopedia you now hold in your hands. And the best thing about it is that this qi and these enchanting aromas and fabulous vibes are available to *everyone*. Every religious tradition has made spiritual use of aromatic plants, because their power is something we have all felt and sensed and been drawn to work with. Every land on Earth is home to aromatic plants, and even the most remote and obscure aromatic plants, once distilled into oil form, can travel anywhere in the world and maintain their aromatic and energetic integrity. No matter your religious, spiritual, or magical tradition, oil magic is open to you.

That said, the effectiveness of your magic depends not only on the quality and choice of your oils but also on the clarity of your intention, the depth of your desire, and your willingness to take action and undergo personal transformation in accord with these. Additionally, I am not a doctor, and nothing in this book should be taken as medical advice (not even, or *especially* not, in chapter 9). Consult a doctor if you experience adverse reactions from using any essential oils.

Throughout this book, for the purpose of ease and readability, I may refer to specific essential oils using the capitalized common name of the plant—you can trust that Lavender refers to the essential oil whereas lavender refers to the plant in fresh or dried form. I may also sometimes use abbreviations such as EO for "essential oil" or FCO for "fractionated coconut oil."

With all that said, I wish you luck and wisdom on your oil magic journey, and all the rewards that come from deepening your spiritual relationship with the natural world. May your life be blessed by the very best plant magic around, and may you feel the full beauty of those blessings in your heart and soul. Happy magic-making and blessed be!

PART I

GREEN WITCHCRAFT IS the art of making magic in harmony with the spirits and forces of nature. A green witch bends the ever-present magic of the natural world to their will, weaving spells and charms from the qi of herbs, spices, trees, flowers, and stones, combined with the power of focus and intention. Essential oil magic is a subset of green witchcraft that utilizes the essential oils of magical plants alongside or instead of fresh or dried plants in spellwork. Working with oils grants a witch access to a wide variety of super-potent plant essences whose physical and subtle energetic properties work together on our bodies, minds, and spirits to support our intentions.

Anyone can be a green witch and practice oil magic. You don't have to choose just one magical specialty—you can use oil magic to enhance every other aspect of your path, from hedgecraft and kitchen witchery to crystal and candle magic. In this part, we'll cover the basic principles of oil magic you'll need to know to get started, from magical theory and ethics to oil history and safety considerations.

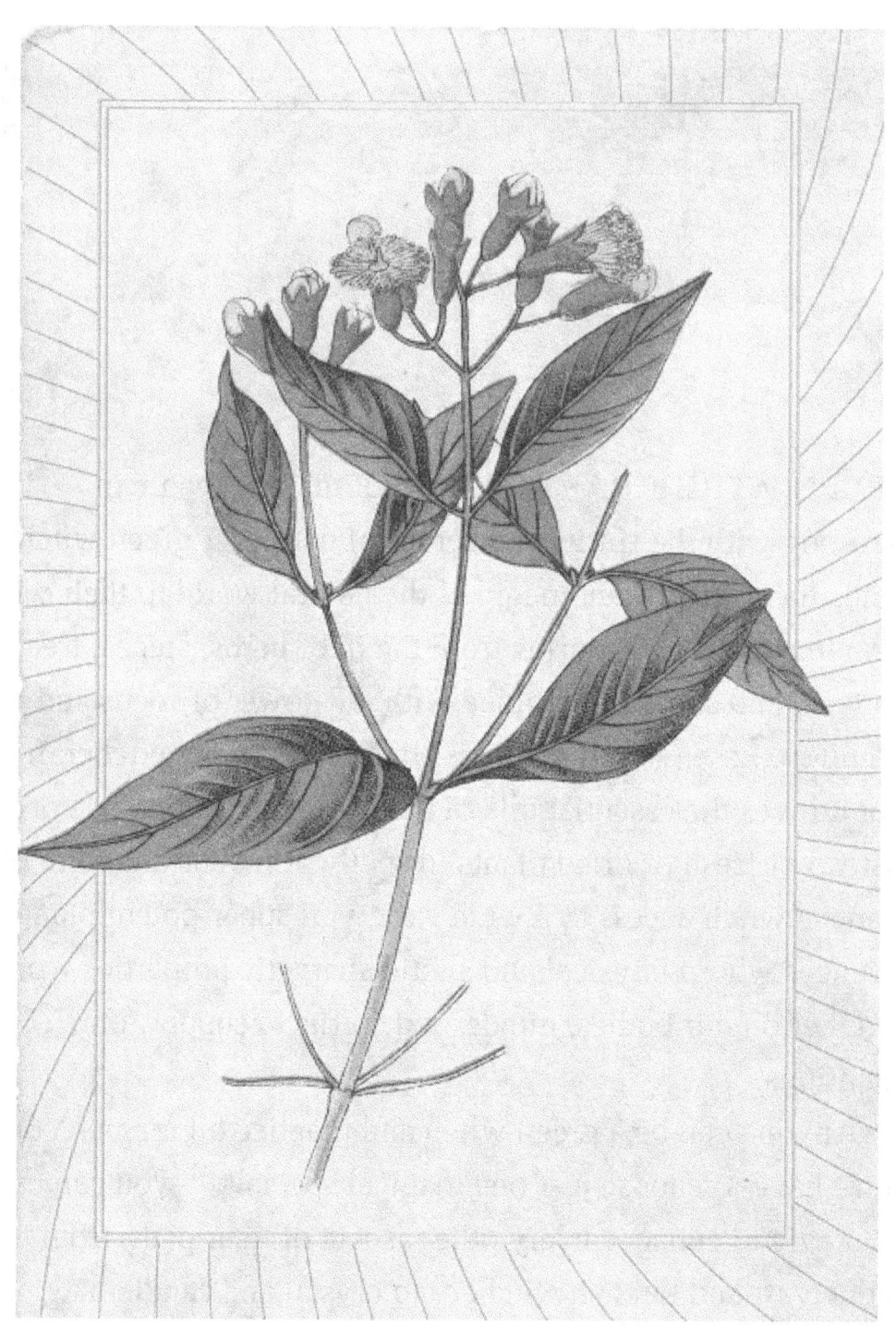

CHAPTER 1

Principles of Magic

BEFORE YOU BEGIN weaving your intentions into reality with the aid of aromatic essences and botanical blends, there are a few practical and theoretical principles to consider. We'll start by covering the basics of green witchcraft and this book's approach in particular. Then, we'll discuss magical morality and I'll offer a few suggestions for keeping your practice ethical. While you *could* just jump right in at that point, remember that your spells may benefit from being performed at a magically appropriate time in a thoughtfully prepared environment. Finally, we'll address visualization, why it is a necessary foundational skill for magic of any kind, and how to improve your technique.

Plant Magic 101

Green witchcraft truly walks the line between magic and science. On the one hand, herbalism and aromatherapy comprise both science and art. By their nature they are difficult to study in a way that appeases modern academics, but each plant and its essential oil has unique physical and chemical properties that affect the human body and mind in ways that are more or less consistent. While the medicinal properties of plants and essential oils are difficult to study scientifically, their spiritual properties are impossible to approach this way. For these, we are guided only by our subtle senses, our intuition, our experiences, and the knowledge our ancestors obtained by those same means.

That said, experience and intuition have proven to be good enough guides that the practice of plant magic is still alive today and is once again growing in popularity. It is one of the most approachable forms of magic and can be practiced by people of any religion—even the Bible is full of references to the spiritual application of plants and oils.

You may be wondering if plant magic is white magic. Such labels are not very useful, as the question of whether a work of magic is good or evil depends on intention and execution. Plant magic is not evil in and of itself. Anything that can heal can also harm, and anything that has power can be perverted, but plants are basically on the side of life and light (quite literally). When we ally ourselves with them by honoring their magic and preserving the strength of their kind, they are quite open to allying themselves with us by lending their power to our intentions. This is especially true if and when our intentions are aligned with the greater purpose of joyful, harmonious, and abundant life on Earth.

The methods presented in this book are inspired by a combination of folk knowledge, research, intuition, and personal experience, and draw from three main approaches.

The first approach is that of herbalism and aromatherapy, which, as fields, generally do their best to approach plant and body chemistry scientifically when possible. For example, I recommend Lavender for divination because it has long been used for relaxation, which is crucial for receiving intuitive guidance.

The second approach is that of sympathetic magic, which makes use of symbolic representations of a goal or intention to manifest that intention in real life. For example, I suggest Rose for protection not because of any compound present in the oil, but because roses protect themselves with thorns. According to the principles of sympathetic magic, the protective power of thorns is carried within the symbol of the rose and can be applied to whatever requires protection.

The third approach is less obvious and sometimes difficult to distinguish from the first two—it is the approach of tuning into the qi or subtle energy and spirit of a plant and its essence to determine its energetic nature and how it wants to be of service. This, I believe, is the approach that led the rose to be associated with romance above all other flowers—there is no known earthly reason *why* it is, it just *is*.

If you find yourself wanting to know more about witchcraft, herbalism, or aromatherapy, there are a multitude of resources on these topics, several of which are suggested in the Resources at the end of this book. To best serve you, the reader, this book focuses specifically on oil magic, which, when it makes use of true essential oils, is the most potent form of plant magic there is.

All in Good Time

You may want to consider the season, moon phase, weekday, hour, or astrological factors when planning and working your magic. Each of these factors can influence and work with or against your magical intentions.

Personally, I have become especially conscious of coordinating my work with the moon cycle, as I have observed that my intentions manifest and come to fruition much more readily when the moon is waxing, and if I try to bring something into my life during the waning moon, it's like swimming against the current. Often, I have found myself working tirelessly toward a goal with no visible progress until finally one day it clicks. That day is usually just after the new moon. When my work requires the energy of a dark or full moon, I tend to give myself about a three-day window of grace to catch it. "Almost" counts in horseshoes, hand grenades, and moon phases.

Magical Ethics

YOU MAY ALREADY have a code of magical ethics that works for you, and that's wonderful! However, if you're new to witchcraft or seeking fresh perspective, here are some basic principles to consider:

- Strive for balance. With any action we take, magical or mundane, it's important to consider the consequences, which often ripple outward considerably. For the greatest likelihood of success and the highest good, the aim of magic should always be to maintain or *restore* balance to the world, not disrupt it. When working with plant magic, this includes the delicate balance of ecosystems: Be sure to source your essential oils from a company that practices sustainable agriculture, gives back to the land, and takes care of their people. When formulating spells and intentions, consider carefully how the desired outcome could create or resolve energetic imbalances. Additionally, make it a habit to give back to the earth as a way of honoring and expressing gratitude for the gifts our mother gives.
- Walk the path of least harm and greatest good. In an ideal world we would do no harm. In this world, however, death is necessary to sustain life, force is often required for self-defense, and ethical consumption is all but impossible. Don't be too hard on yourself, but do aim to make choices that lift others up, put power in the

hands of good people, and give back to the earth. Walking the path of the greatest good also means taking care of yourself so that you can continue to be of greater service to the world. The more you are rooted in love, the easier this is to do.

✦ Seek power from within. Seeking power over others leads to resentment on all sides. Furthermore, the illusion of having power over others is a distraction from all that you can accomplish by gaining mastery over yourself. Focus instead on cultivating power from within and mastering your own thoughts and behaviors. As you step into the full power of who you are meant to be, your world will begin to shape itself accordingly. Trying to force change on your external reality without transforming your inner reality is like trying to change the shape of a shadow without moving the light source or altering the form that casts it. Your qi is the light and your actions are the form.

The seasons can also influence our magic and personal energy. The best illustration of this is the Wheel of the Year, which divides the solar year into eight sections by season, separated by the solstices (winter and summer), the equinoxes (spring and autumn), and days known as the cross-quarters. Winter Solstice marks the longest night and shortest day; it is both the heart of darkness and the rebirth of the Sun, and is a good time for rest, reflection, and setting intentions. Imbolc (February 1st in the Northern Hemisphere) encourages the returning light and the thawing of winter. It is a good time for cleansing and purification, and for planting seeds, both literally and metaphorically. By Spring Equinox, night and day are equal and warmth returns to the earth. This is the most fertile time, and is a good time to let intentions gain momentum, especially surrounding love. Beltane (May 1st) celebrates the impending summer. It is super-powered for manifestation and its energy is highly sexual. Summer Solstice marks the longest day and the shortest night. It is the high point of the year's energy, and is a ripe time for creativity and rapid manifestation. By Lammas (August 1st, the first harvest festival), it's time to start thinking about tying up loose ends and putting the fruits of your creative energy in order. At Autumn Equinox, day and night are equal again. This is the time to reap what you sowed and enjoy it with gratitude. Samhain (November 1st) marks the fading of the light into darkness and is the festival of death and endings. This is a time to release and bury anything that has not manifested during the year, and to honor losses and failures for their lessons. Take this time to reflect, be grateful, and connect with your ancestors and departed loved ones.

The seven days of the week are named for the seven "planets" of classical astrology, so you may wish to take advantage of the correspondences that exist there (see here). For example, if you are working love magic, which is ruled by Venus, in addition to choosing oils ruled by Venus (see chapter 6) you may also wish to work the spell on a Friday if it is convenient. This can be a nice "extra," but will not make or break a spell.

I am not too choosy about specific hours of the day, but if you want to work with certain celestial or planetary energies, their power may peak at very specific times, and that may be something you wish to take advantage of. At the very least, I do find that some spells are better worked by moonlight and some in the light of day: You may want to harness the sun's power to enhance confidence and positivity, or the moon's fullness to inspire love and enchantment.

Location, Location, Location

It is important to work magic in an environment that is conducive to focus and imagination (visualization). Usually this means a peaceful place free of clutter and distractions. I like working magic outside when I can, with the trees, roses, and the heavens as my witnesses, but this is not always practical.

Speaking of practicality, with oil magic, you will want to work someplace where it would not be a huge problem if you have a little spill. If you are someone who does most of your magical work at an altar, simply place a dish on your altar to catch any spills and carry on as usual.

For small everyday spells, however, you need not stand on ceremony. Much magic, including many of the suggestions found in later chapters of this book, can be done with nothing more than small tools you can carry in your purse or pocket (thank you, roller bottles!). In these cases, your working environment is your own body and mind. Because essential oils are natural allies for cleansing the body and mind, you can use them to help cultivate within yourself an ideal environment for magical practice. However, allowing toxins and energetic clutter into your body and mind when working with essential oils is much like carrying crystals to manifest abundance while complaining about scarcity. Your body *is* your temple—it is the place from which you participate in all acts of worship, magic, creation, gratitude, love, and joy. Care for your body as a home worthy of your human spirit like you would care for a temple as a home worthy of a deity, and you will always have a good place to work magic.

Planning & Preparing

Before using oils topically, be sure to perform patch tests (see here), which can reveal potential sensitivities and spare you a good deal of irritation—literally. Additionally, review general essential oil safety in chapter 4 and any oil-specific precautions in chapter 6.

Beyond that, it is always a good idea to prepare for a magical working by clearing the mind. Clear mental clutter by brain dumping in a journal, drinking water, and taking a few deep breaths. Then, take a moment to ground and center yourself.

You may also wish to cleanse your body before working. Showers not only cleanse the body but also clear the mind and purify energy. Add a few drops of pure Eucalyptus, Rosemary, Lemon, Lavender, or Peppermint, or a combination thereof, to your shower floor to assist energy cleansing.

As you work more closely with the magic of the natural world, you may find that you have a stronger connection to it when you consume more whole foods, fewer processed foods, and fewer synthetic products. That said, it's not what goes into someone's mouth that defiles them, but what comes out of it, so you do you. You can also deepen your relationship with nature by spending more time outdoors, learning your local flora, or tending to some plants of your own.

Visualization

Visualization is an important skill for any type of magic, and you will be called upon to use it many times throughout this book. Proper visualization depends on you knowing, understanding, and imagining your intended outcome with precision and clarity. If you do not *know* what you want, you cannot even begin to manifest it. If you do not *understand* which aspects of your desire are important, you may manifest the trappings without the core. And if you cannot *imagine* what you want, how will you recognize it when it appears?

Despite the name, visualization is not just about visual imagery—all the senses can participate in visualization. More important than sight or sound is the internal and emotional *feeling* surrounding your goal. It's good to picture bigger numbers in your bank account or the partner of your dreams by your side, but it's even better to tune in to the somatic and emotional feelings of abundance, love, and security. Tune in to the feelings you want to create, and they will be that much easier to recognize later.

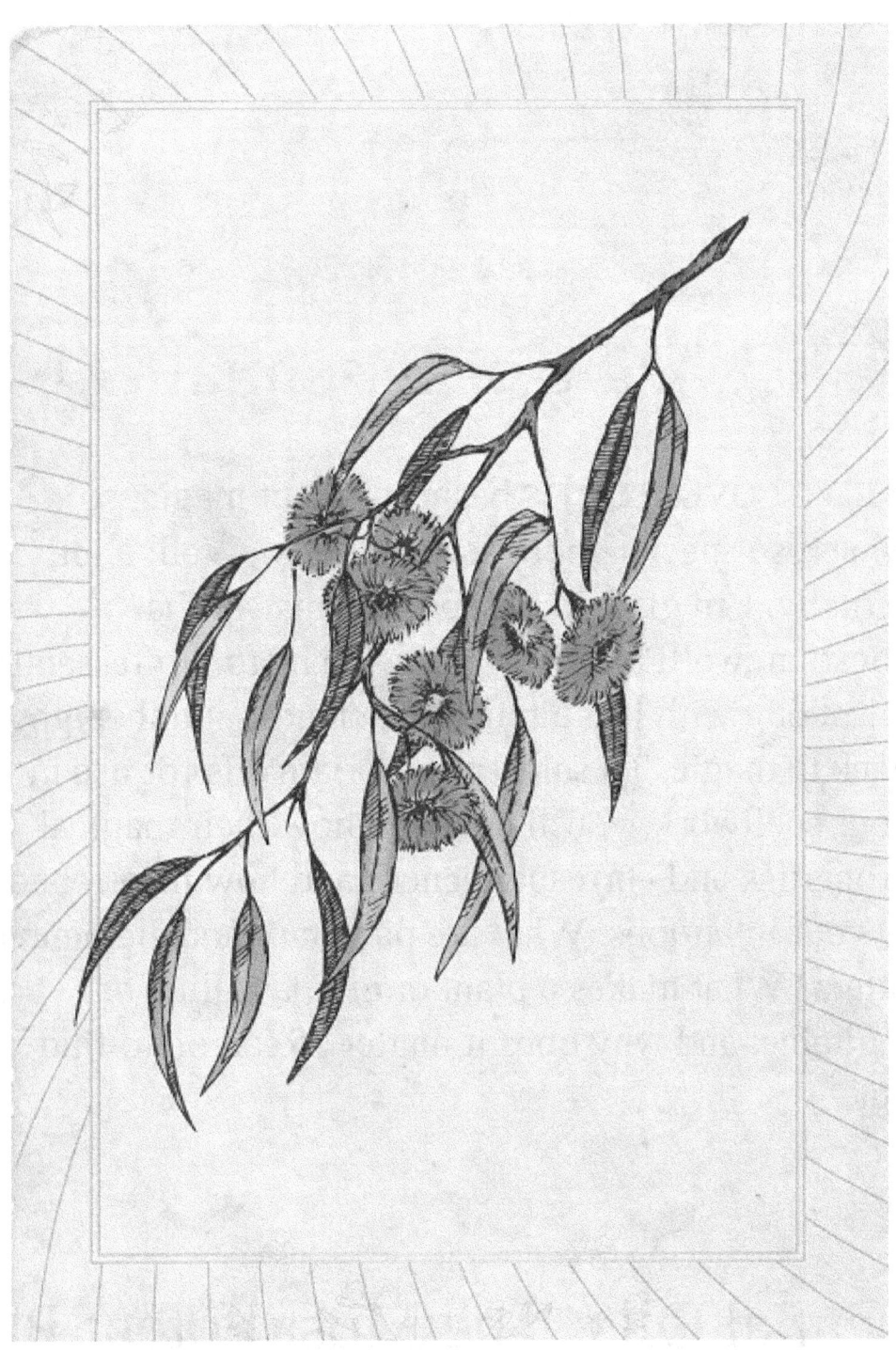

CHAPTER 2

The Magic of Essential Oils

WE'VE COVERED THE basics of plant magic, so what's so special about essential oils? Well, a lot, actually. I'm glad you asked! To answer that question, we'll briefly explore the history of essential oils along with just a touch of science, and then go back to magic. To select appropriate oils for use in your spellwork, you'll need to know their magical properties and correspondences and how they relate to your intentions. What are planetary and elemental rulers? What makes a plant or oil masculine or feminine, and why does it matter? Read on to find out.

Essential Oils: The Most Potent Plant Magic

You may know of essential oils as something used in spas, natural personal care products, and eco-friendly household cleaners. Although these are all great uses for them, the world of essential oils is full of so much more possibility! Not only are they invaluable everyday assets for everything from supporting your body's natural immune response to helping you deal with difficult emotions, but they are also potent magical allies that can empower your spells, transform your potions, and charge up your charms.

Essential oils are the most potent form of plant magic. How can this be? An essential oil is the distilled or extracted aromatic *essence* of a given plant. The compounds that make a plant what it is, that make a plant do what it does, are contained within that plant's essential oil. A single essential oil distilled from a single species of plant can contain a multitude of chemical compounds, and these compounds have physical effects on the body and mind that can be harnessed through the practices of herbalism and aromatherapy. Furthermore, the qi, or spiritual essence, of a plant is preserved in the proper distillation of its essential oil, which makes high-quality essential oils . . . well, *essential* to the apothecary of any witch worth their salt.

Traditional plant magic requires access to the fresh plant for greatest potency, as essential oils dissipate over time in dried specimens. That's why your dried herbs and spices only last a year at most and never smell as strong as when you first open them. (For spicing up soups and spells, it's the oils contained within the plant that you really want anyway.) With proper distillation and storage, most essential oils can last for years, if not forever; although once you see how fun and easy they are to use and how effective they are at what they do, you'll have more trouble keeping them in stock than using them up.

The variety of applications is endless: Essential oils can be diffused to alter the energy of a space and those who inhabit it; they can be made into magical sprays, salves, balms, and perfumes; they can be blended into bath salts, massage oils, and body butters; and specially-labeled dietary essential oils can even be incorporated into your culinary exploits. By nature, essential oils are easy to use, store, transport, and preserve, which means they make it possible for anyone to easily and conveniently access a wider, more shelf-stable, and more potent variety of plant magic than could ever be possible with fresh or dried plant matter.

With essential oils in your magical toolkit, you'll have a whole new world of plant magic at your fingertips—and what a wonderful world it is!

History of Oil Magic

Humans have been enjoying the benefits of essential oils for as long as we have walked this earth. When you breathe in the fresh air of a forest or stop to smell the roses, you inhale essential oils. When you drink mint tea or cook with fresh rosemary, you consume essential oils. As society grows more and more separate from nature and the lifestyles of our ancestors, we have had to employ ingenuity and technology to bring the magic and medicine of plants and their enchanting aromas back into our lives.

In ancient times, there was no distinction between magical healing and medicine. As such, the ancient uses of aromatic plants and their essences can be thought of as magical, medicinal, or both. In any case, there is evidence of aromatic plants being combined with fatty oils (e.g., olive, sesame) to create ointments by ca. 5000 BCE. These would have been created with direct infusion techniques such as enfleurage or heated infusion. Other early methods of aromatherapy may have included steam diffusion by simmering herbs and resins in water and then inhaling or soaking up the aromatic steam.

The oldest known still, a terra cotta model from the Indus Valley, dates back to the beginning of the Bronze Age (ca. 3000 BCE). Distillation made essential oils available in a much more potent and user-friendly form, similar to what we use today. The *Ebers Papyrus*, which dates back to the 1500s BCE but is thought to have been copied from earlier texts, contains 877 remedies, many of which call for essential oils or their botanical counterparts. By ca. 1157 BCE, aromatic oils and ointments were so integral to daily life that Egyptian craftsmen under Pharaoh Ramesses III went on the first-ever recorded labor strike, citing "no ointment" among their complaints.

Not just for the living, oils and resins such as myrrh and juniper were used to prepare the dead for the afterlife as part of the Egyptian embalming process ca. 3200 BCE. Later, frankincense oil was considered important enough to be carried into the afterlife by a pharaoh: The tomb of Tutankhamun (dated to ca. 1300s BCE) was found to contain alabaster jars filled with the stuff.

Over time, the use of essential oils spread from the Middle East to Greece, Rome, and the rest of Europe. By 400 BCE, the Greek physician Hippocrates, considered the father of medicine, claimed that the key to good health began with a daily aromatic bath and massage.

Beyond health and wellness, the Bible contains a multitude of references to the use of essential oils for spiritual purposes (ca. 1600 BCE to 85 CE). Frankincense and myrrh were among the gifts to the infant Jesus, and besides their practical uses, frankincense was a symbol of divinity, and myrrh a symbol of death and eternal life. Though these oils were (and to some extent still are) costly, they were not just for royalty: Jen O'Sullivan notes in her book *The Essential Oil Truth* that Rome reportedly used 2,800 tons of frankincense and 500 tons of myrrh annually ca. 100 BCE. Speaking of royalty, Cleopatra (69 to 30 BCE) was known for her seductive perfume blends and for taking milk baths with oils of Jasmine, Rose, and Myrrh to enhance her beauty.

In the 1200s CE, Islamic Andalusian polymath Ibn al-Baitar created a pharmacopoeia, or pharmaceutical encyclopedia, that includes many essential oils and their uses as well as the oldest written instructions for distillation. The coronation ceremony of the British monarch includes an anointing rite that has used the same oil recipe since 1626, one that includes Rose, Neroli, Jasmine, and Cinnamon in a base of olive and sesame oils.

Though essential oils never fell out of use, more recent centuries treated them as mere perfume. Magic and healing took a back seat to science and cosmetics as the modern age progressed. In 1937, however, Dr. René-Maurice Gattefossé coined the concept of aromatherapy as its own discipline after rediscovering the healing potential of lavender oil in a lab accident. Madame Marguerite Maury and Dr. Jean Valnet continued to research, practice, and promote aromatherapy, which gained traction in the US in the late 1980s and early 1990s and has continued to grow in popularity ever since.

What Makes Oils Magical

All true essential oils are magical, as all plants possess magic, although some are more famous than others. Essential oils are different from plant matter in that they are volatile. Their molecules have such low atomic mass that they rise readily into the air, where we can inhale them, and are so small that they can easily pass through cell walls and the blood-brain barrier.

Each essential oil has its own unique qi, chemical constituents, and stimulating aroma. All three of these are fundamental elements of the magic of essential oils.

The qi is what we interact with magically. It is the subtle energy of the plant to which you attune, and that harmonizes with your intention. Books can give you a general sense of the qi of a plant or oil, but every specimen of a plant and every batch of an oil will have slightly different qi depending on its life story. Qi defies total explanation in both the general and specific senses. To interact with it with any sort of intentionality, you must learn to sense it directly. This process will be discussed in the section on attunement in chapter 5.

The chemical constituents are what we actually inhale or absorb when we use essential oils topically, aromatically, or internally, whereas the aroma is the olfactory experience of those constituents. If you would like to learn more about the specific constituents of essential oils and the effects they have on the body, the Resources section at the end of this book contains suggestions for further reading.

The third component is aroma. Have you ever smelled something and felt immediately transported to a particular memory of a person or place? When we inhale essential oils, the constituent compounds are transported by the olfactory system directly to the emotional center of the brain, activating memories and associated emotions. Because of this, aroma becomes a tool for mindfulness and emotional regulation. This is a crucial component of oil magic.

Cultivating Respect

AS YOU BEGIN to research more about essential oils beyond this book, you may notice a lot of fear around these powerful bottles of plant magic, but I don't think that fear is necessary. Instead, I propose we cultivate a healthy *respect* for the plants and oils we harness for our purposes, and seek to understand them more deeply so that our experiences with them may be entirely positive.

Truth be told, our comfortable lives are so separated from nature that we are able to romanticize nature without recognizing its ability to cause harm. It's easy to think that because essential oils are natural, they are harmless. This is not true. Nature is not for or against us—it's trying to *survive*, and if we get in the way of that, or misunderstand it, we may get hurt. For example, certain oils like lemon are considered "phototoxic." What this really means is that these fruits have evolved to be able to magnify the sunlight they absorb within themselves, affording them the ability to grow and ripen more efficiently. However, when we apply these oils to our skin, we absorb this ability, and the sunlight that hits our skin is magnified as well. Instead of ripening, we burn, sometimes to the extreme. But you need not fear citrus oils. Merely learn to respect them and harness their power appropriately.

Then, there are studies that claim certain oils cause seizures, or something similarly horrifying. These studies are often based on use of isolated constituents and extreme dosages. Five milliliters may be a small amount of milk to drink, but if someone drinks five milliliters of essential oil, it is safe to say that they have taken absolutely zero time to understand how essential oils work. If you understand that essential oils are powerful, concentrated plant medicine dispensed by the drop, you are not in danger of drinking entire bottles of the stuff and need not fear.

I cannot overstate this: *Do your own research*. Think critically. Don't make assumptions. Dive deep, ask questions, don't drink entire bottles of essential oil, and keep them out of reach of children, and you need not be afraid. When used properly and with due respect, essential oils are quite safe and can be very helpful.

Here are a few principles of healthy respect for plant magic:

- What is good for the plant may be helpful or harmful to you depending on the circumstances. Every person is different and will react differently to every oil.
- If a little is good, more is *not* always better. Essential oils are very concentrated, and there *can* be too much of a good thing.
- Kids are more sensitive than adults. Babies are very sensitive. Pets are a different animal entirely—literally.
- Always read the label and take package directions to heart.
- Do not assume that everyone who uses essential oils knows what they're talking about. Just because your friend does it doesn't make it a good idea. Just because your friend says it's toxic doesn't make it so.
- Research an oil before patch testing it and pay attention to how you feel after.

- Trust your intuition but verify when possible. If your gut leads you to a particular oil, research it and try it out.

Along with respecting the *power* of plants, we must also cultivate a respect for their right to go on living as more than an ingredient in our oil apothecaries. This means researching the sourcing and farming practices of the companies we purchase from. Oils such as Indian Sandalwood and Palo Santo can be difficult to source ethically and sustainably. Australian Sandalwood and Royal Hawaiian Sandalwood are sustainable alternatives to Indian Sandalwood, and Palo Santo oil, which is distilled only from naturally fallen branches, is available if you care to search for it. Cultivate respect for these and other beloved plants before seeking to harness their powers, and you are much less likely to end up in hot water with them.

Properties & Correspondences

Essential oils are the chemical and spiritual essences of aromatic plants, and plants are complex living things. As such, there are no hard and fast rules surrounding the magical uses of plants or their essential oils. Intuition and experience will be your best guides, but until you have the experience to guide your intuition, you must have something to go on and somewhere to start. That's where magical correspondences and the other information found in this book can help you. Everything from gender polarity and planetary rulers to elemental associations and herb lore can influence what magical intentions and purposes an oil is best suited for. Look at the oil profiles in chapter 6 to guide your selections as you alter the spells in this book for personal use and write your own.

When researching and selecting oils you wish to use, pay attention to the scientific (Latin) names of the plants the oils are distilled from. It may surprise you to know that *Matricaria chamomilla* and *Chamaemelum nobile* are two different plants that both go by the common name of chamomile. Ravensara (*Ravensara aromatica*) and Ravintsara (*Cinnamomum camphora*) are two separate oils that are quite different and just as easy to confuse by name. Scientific names are useful for knowing exactly what botanical you're using, but in addition to these and common names, some plants also have magical names or folk names that reveal something of their energetic character or lore, such as "Dew of the Sea" for rosemary or "Devil Plant" for basil.

Once you know precisely what essences you're dealing with, you can look up and research their magical properties and correspondences in chapter 6 to gain understanding and inspiration for incorporating them into your witchcraft. You can then make informed substitutions and use the spells and blends in chapters 7 to 11 as jumping-off points for creating your own spells and blends.

Polarity

In magical tradition, things are thought of as masculine or feminine based on whether their magical action is active or receptive. Fire, air, wands, swords, and herbs such as basil and juniper are traditionally thought to have more active and aggressive (yang) natures and are classified as masculine. Earth, water, discs, cups, and herbs such as cardamom and jasmine are traditionally thought to have more receptive and magnetic (yin) natures and are therefore classified as feminine.

In the most general sense, masculine herbs and oils are well suited for vitality, protection, purification, courage, and success magic, whereas feminine herbs and oils are better suited to spells for fertility, abundance, love, divination, and healing. That said, a traditionally masculine herb that encourages passion may be useful in love magic with other feminine herbs, and a traditionally feminine herb that attracts wealth may be useful in spells for success. Additionally, the specific nature of most plants is more complex than this dichotomy. For example, basil is associated not just with luck and protection but also with money and love. Gender polarity is one way to understand the energetic action of a plant ally, but do not place too much stock in this dimension alone. You risk oversimplifying the complex nature of individual oils, which each have a wide variety of magical applications that may or may not be confined to the territory traditionally corresponding to their polarities.

Magical Intentions

Each plant ally and its essential oil are best suited to a particular range of intentions, many of which will be described in the oil profiles in chapter 6. The spells in this book are divided into five categories based on general intention: protection, love, healing, wealth, and divination. Most spells and specific intentions can be placed in one of these categories.

Protection magic includes banishing, energy clearing, boundary setting, cloaking, luck spells, and blessings. These sorts of spells can help protect your personal energy, your loved ones, your home, and your possessions.

Love magic starts with enhancing self-love and self-esteem, which in turn boosts personal magnetism and attractiveness. It also includes magic designed to smooth, sweeten, or bless relationships of all kinds, as well as spells for passion and commitment.

Healing magic is best used to supplement the usual methods of achieving and maintaining wellness. This book includes spells for encouraging and supporting the body's natural healing process, for practicing self-care and staying motivated, and to aid in spiritual and emotional healing.

Wealth magic includes manifestation and prosperity spells. Manifestation can be used for many things besides money, such as a happy home or fulfilling employment, just as personal wealth is measured by more than solely dollars.

Divination magic includes spirit communication, spells for boosting intuition and clarity, blessings and enchantments for divinatory tools, and anything that helps you find the answers you seek.

Planetary Rulers

The seven planets of classical astrology are each assigned particular spheres of influence. Regardless of whether or not you make astrology a part of your practice, the seven "planets" (really five planets and two luminaries, the Sun and Moon) can serve as shorthand for their domains of influence. That is to say, a plant's planetary ruler can tell you what sort of magical intentions that plant and its oil are well suited for.

Oils from plants ruled by the Sun are well suited to spells for good luck, success, confidence, and positivity. Moon-ruled oils can aid with divination, intuition, inner work (e.g., shadow work), transformation, and inspiration. Mars rules courage, willpower and strength, justice, defense, and virility. Mercury has dominion over communication and travel, creativity and inspiration, wisdom and learning, and adaptation. Jupiter governs matters of power and influence, business, prosperity, well-being, luck, and success. If a plant is ruled by Venus, you can bet that it would be appropriate to use in love and glamour spells as well as magic for beauty, luxury, and sensual pleasures. Finally, Saturn governs hard work, life lessons, structure, discipline, and endings that make way for new beginnings.

Elemental Rulers

Western occultism uses a system of four primary elements—earth, air, fire, and water—plus the fifth element of spirit. Spirit is generally considered to be woven throughout the other four and is immaterial. The other four elements are material but are associated with metaphysical and immaterial qualities and characteristics.

Earth is the foundation and governs material resources, wealth and prosperity, security and stability, home, family, fertility, and ancestral work. Its energy is abundant and grounding. Air rules communication, analytical and rational thought, intellect, inspiration, divination, and freedom. Its energy is expansive and clarifying. Fire governs passion, courage, creativity, power, purification, and protection, and is motivational and energizing by nature. Water rules emotions and relationships, peace, wellness, and intuition, and its energy is cleansing, restorative, and loving.

Like gender and planetary correspondences, elemental correspondences can help you select the appropriate ingredients for your spells, charms, and potions.

Colors

It would be a stretch to associate colors with oils directly in any magical sense, since each plant has its own color given by nature and many plants and oils are well suited to a diversity of magical intentions. However, it cannot be denied that colors have an almost universal symbolic language that can be used to enhance spellwork.

This color symbolism can be applied when choosing candles, cloth, ink, crystals, clothing and jewelry, and more to include in your magical workings. Generally, red is associated with passion, lust, vigor, and blood mysteries; pink with love, beauty, and wellness; orange with creativity, inspiration, and adventure; yellow with friendship, joy, luck, happiness, and abundance; green with health, fertility, and finances; blue with peace, communication, and wisdom; purple with intuition, spirituality, and divination; brown with stability, roots, and grounding; black with protection; and white with purity, clarity, cleansing, and divinity. Gold is solar and silver is lunar and celestial. White or uncolored material (such as naturally yellow beeswax) can be used for any intention in place of a specific color.

PART II

ESSENTIAL OILS ARE magical and awesome, we get it, but how can we bring this oily plant magic into our lives and put it into practice for ourselves? In this part, myth and history become your everyday magical reality as we jump out of the sarcophagus of theory and into the cauldron of practice. What makes some oils better than others, and why does it matter? Where can you buy good ones? Once you have them, how do you store them, and what on earth do you do with them? What's a blend and how do you make one, or should you buy them? Does it matter what carrier oils you use? What if you don't have a particular oil? Read on for the answers to all these questions and more.

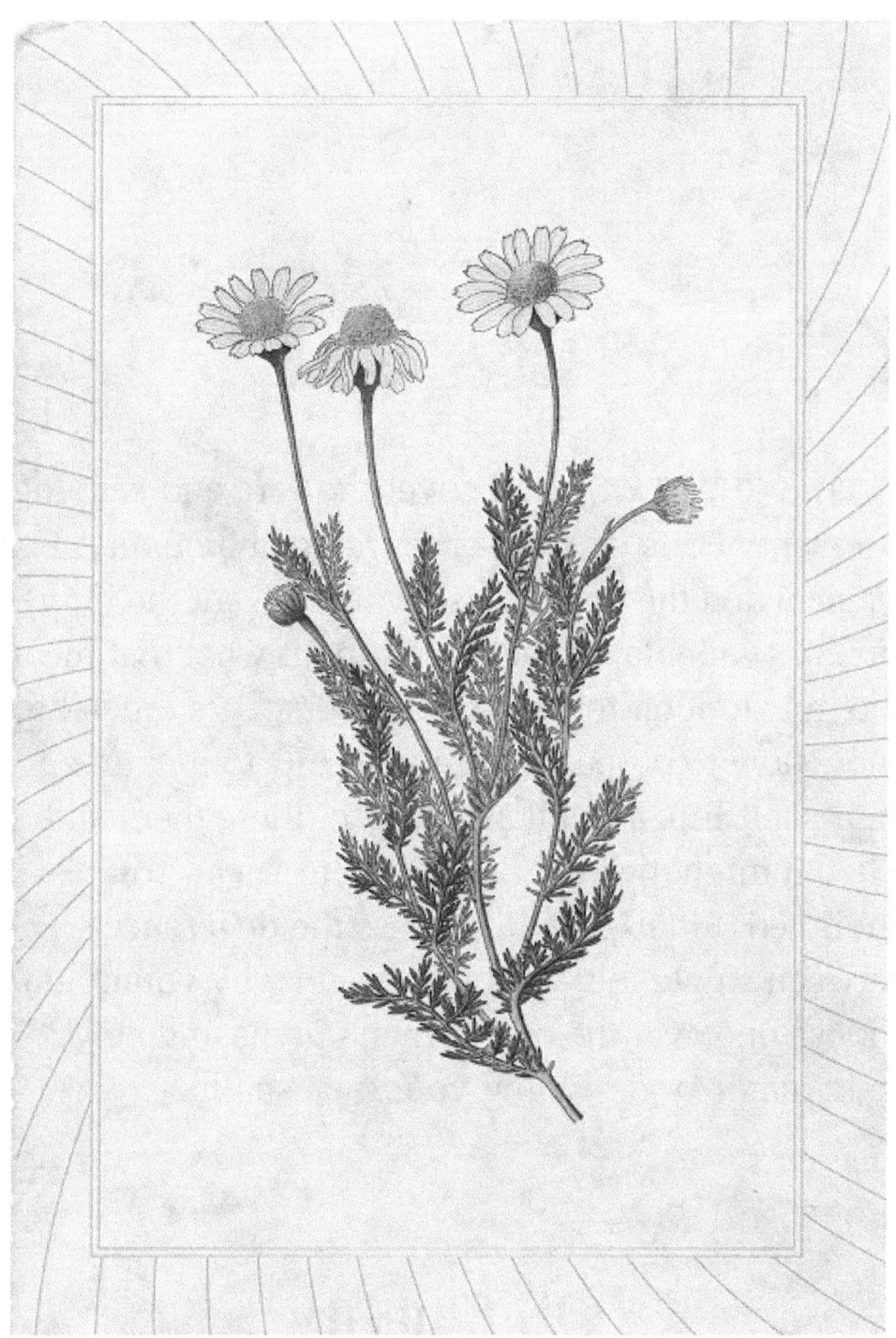

CHAPTER 3

On Essential Oils

IN THIS CHAPTER, we'll cover the care and keeping of essential oils, as well as sourcing and quality. For magical and therapeutic use, you *do* want the highest quality available, so we'll talk about what that means and how to look for it. And of course, it's crucial to know how to properly store your oils to maximize their shelf life, as well as when to dilute them and when it might be better to use them "neat," or undiluted. Finally, we'll discuss the difference between single oils and blends, and why you might choose one over the other when purchasing new plant magic or designing your own spells.

Oil Quality

Not all essential oils are created equal. In fact, not all bottles labeled "100% pure essential oil" are even essential oil. To bear that label, a bottle need only contain 5 percent essential oil by volume! This is because, in the United States, essential oils are classified by the Food and Drug Administration as cosmetics and are not regulated. Anyone can slap some smelly stuff into a bottle, label it "essential oil," and sell it as such, unless someone else goes out of their way to prove that it doesn't contain a minimum of 5 percent essential oil by volume.

AFNOR (*Association Française de Normalisation*) is a French organization that sets standards for constituent levels in true unadulterated oils. The idea is that if an oil is tested, it should have the correct chemical constituents in the correct amounts to meet AFNOR standards. Ideally, if an essential oil is adulterated, the amounts will not be correct and constituents that should not be present will be detected. AFNOR standards can help prevent adulteration (assuming a company voluntarily submits their oils for testing, since essential oils are not required to meet AFNOR standards to be sold in the US), but they can't do much about synthetic oils. In fact, AFNOR standards provide a perfect recipe for what compounds to synthesize and in what ratios so as to make a synthetic "essential oil." You might think, "Well, if it meets AFNOR standards, then what could be wrong with it?" and I used to think the same thing. But as it turns out, the answer is "plenty."

For one, synthetic constituents can be completely different isomers of a given molecule than those produced naturally by the source plant. This means that a plant and a chemist can generate molecules with the same name and molecular formula but with different structures, properties, and effects on the body.

For another, no essential oil has ever been comprehensively analyzed. Each essential oil contains a multitude of chemical constituents, but only the ones appearing in the highest percentages have been analyzed and identified. However, the unidentified trace components of high-quality essential oils may make a significant difference in the effects and properties of the whole oil. Someone in a lab may synthesize unnatural isomers of the compounds present in lavender oil, combine them in the AFNOR standard quantities, and have something that passes AFNOR standards yet is wholly different from a properly distilled natural lavender oil. It's important to know, too, that if you are interested in magical use, synthetic oils will certainly not possess the qi of the source plant.

How Essential Oils Are Produced

TECHNICALLY, THE TERM "essential oil" refers only to the volatile compounds that can be steam distilled from fresh plant matter. Fresh plant matter is placed in a distillation apparatus over boiling water, and the steam from the water rises through the plant matter, bringing the volatile compounds out of the plant matter. Then, the steam and gaseous oils are condensed into liquid as they are cooled, the oil separates from the water, and voilà! You have essential oil.

However, steam distillation is not possible for certain oils. Many of Jasmine's crucial constituents are destroyed by heat, so Jasmine is produced as an absolute. Instead of steam, absolutes are extracted with chemical solvents, and some of the solvents inevitably remain in the finished absolute. For this reason, though aromatic and indubitably magical, absolutes are generally not considered appropriate for topical or internal use. CO_2 extractions are an alternative to absolutes using carbon dioxide, which does not leave residual contaminants behind.

Citrus peel oils also lose constituents to steam, but they are so rich in oil that they can be cold-pressed. Cold expression leaves no chemical residue and preserves the complete oil profile. However, the components of oils like Lemon, Lime, and Bergamot that are destroyed by steam distillation are those that make them phototoxic, so depending on your desired usage, you may prefer steam-distilled citrus oils (often labeled as furocoumarin-free, FCF, or bergapten-free).

To reduce costs and increase profit margins, many companies will perform a first distillation with steam, and then follow up with further distillations using chemical solvents. This produces a more finished product that can be sold at a lower cost, but it is of a much lower quality than a pure steam distillation, and like absolutes, these oils will not be pure. Other cost-cutting practices include stretching plant-derived oils with synthetic compounds, diluting essential oils with carrier oil or alcohol, adding or substituting similar but less costly oils (such as selling Lavandin as Lavender, Cassia as Cinnamon, or using less-desirable species of Frankincense). When a company with rigorous quality standards rejects a batch of oil, less scrupulous companies will sometimes buy the reject batch from the supplier, alter it (or not), bottle it, and sell it themselves. With essential oils, as with many things, you get what you pay for.

Assuming that what's in your bottle is actually 100 percent pure and plant-derived, you also want oils that have been properly grown, harvested, and distilled. Everything from the climate to the mineral content of the soil can affect the volatile compounds present in the source plant, and many plants must be harvested at specific times of day for the highest concentration of beneficial compounds. Then, each plant must be distilled at very specific sets of times and temperatures so as to extract the greatest number of constituents without destroying any in the process.

Finally, especially where magical use is concerned, it is best to use oils distilled from plants that were sown, tended, harvested, distilled, and bottled with love, care, and positive intent. Such an oil will have much better qi than one that is produced solely for profit.

Buying Oils

The lack of external regulation can make it difficult to tell the quality of an oil before purchasing it and testing it yourself, but there are things you can look for when shopping for high-quality essential oils.

Your first clue is price. More expensive does not always mean better, but if it seems too good to be true, it probably is. Given the amount of time, care, technology, and plant matter that goes into growing, harvesting, distilling, testing, bottling, and distributing a high-quality oil, it's understandable that they're not cheap. If an oil's price seems cheap, it is probably diluted, adulterated, fractionated, synthetic, or unsustainable.

Another thing to look for when buying oils is transparency in the growing, harvesting, distillation, and testing processes from the company you're considering, as well as the "right" answers to a few questions about their sources, methods, and standards. You may be able to find some information on their website, but often you will have better luck calling or emailing the company. Jen O'Sullivan has a fantastic and very thorough list of 22 questions to ask essential oil companies and a detailed explanation of the answers to look for in her book *The Essential Oil Truth: The Facts without the Hype*. Here are a few questions to get you started in your investigation of potential essential oil suppliers (you want a "yes" to all of these before you commit to a purchase):

- Do they distill their own oils (as opposed to buying them)?
- Do they own any of their own farms? Can you visit them?
- Do they test every batch for purity with third-party labs?
- Are their oils safe to ingest (within reason)?
- Are they invested in sustainability and giving back?

Storage

Pure, high-quality essential oils should last at least two years if stored properly in a cool, dark place away from children and animals; many can last for much longer, although many experts suggest replacing opened oils every three years. Oils that have been diluted with a carrier oil will have the shelf life of the carrier oil, which is usually much shorter. If the look or smell of an oil has changed from when you first opened it, that's a good indication not to use it.

Keeping your bottles tightly sealed is important to prevent oxidation. Oxidation changes the chemistry of an oil, so using an oxidized essential oil can have unexpected, unpredictable, and unwanted effects. Only break the seal on a bottle you are ready to use and recap your bottles quickly after opening them to limit oxygen exposure. Less headroom is better, so if you've used a lot of an oil, you may wish to transfer it to a smaller bottle where it will have less headroom and therefore less oxygen.

Another threat to your precious oils is ultraviolet radiation, or light. This is why oils are generally sold in dark-colored bottles (amber is best). The bottles must be glass or stainless steel, because essential oils can degrade plastic containers over time, ruining both container and oil. I sometimes use clear, or colorless, glass roller bottles, but will generally store those in my purse or in another place where light cannot reach them.

Heat is also damaging to oils (and some of them are flammable), so definitely keep them away from any heat sources. If you live in a warm climate, be sure not to store them in your car. You can extend the shelf life of many oils by keeping them in the refrigerator.

Finally, if you have pets or kids, be sure to store your oils safely out of their reach. Besides being too costly to risk spilling, in the wrong hands, essential oils can be the wrong kind of powerful.

Neat versus Diluted

There are many ways to use essential oils, and not all essential oil users agree on what is appropriate or responsible. Neat use of undiluted oils is one such topic of contention. On the one hand, millions of people regularly apply neat, or undiluted, oils to their skin without ever having any issue at all. On the other hand, some oils known as "hot oils" can be irritants and cause a reaction in some people when used neat. Additionally, some people develop dermal sensitivities to certain oils after extended periods of successful use, and the consensus is that the higher the frequency of use and the higher the concentration—neat being 100 percent concentrated—the higher the risk of sensitization.

Sensitization is the body's way of saying, "enough is enough!" Most people will probably not become sensitized to their favorite oils, but anyone can be at any time without warning, and dilution reduces the risk of sensitization. Be especially mindful with broken skin, as it is more prone to sensitizing.

So, can you use your oils neat? Probably, in most cases, although hot oils such as Cinnamon and Oregano should pretty much always be diluted, and certain oils like Vetiver and Lemongrass are considered at higher risk for sensitization. Ask yourself if it's more important for you to use your oils neat than it is for you to reduce your risk of sensitization. Is your reason for wanting to use an oil neat merely one of convenience? The spells in this book make use of dispersed or diluted oils by means of diffuser blends, roller bottles, bath bombs, massage oils, and more, so neat use will not be necessary to follow along.

Personally, I use oils neat sometimes, but not daily, and certainly not the same oils neat daily. I can usually get just as much benefit from a diluted oil, and I would be inconsolable if I could no longer use my beloved Frankincense, Vetiver, or Black Spruce. The main thing is to know about the individual oils you are working with and the risks you are taking, so that you can make informed decisions for yourself. And finally, however you decide to *use* your oils, you never want to purchase prediluted oils, unless you are certain of the quality and intend to *use* them up quickly; essential oils do not go rancid, but carrier oils do, and you don't want your oils to go to waste.

Single Oils versus Blends

When purchasing essential oils, you have the option to purchase either single oils or blends. Neither is better than the other. I personally have both types in my collection.

A single oil is the essence of a single species of plant, and ideally it is single origin as well. If you are planning to build a versatile apothecary and don't mind spending a little extra to have more options and more control, you will probably want to focus on building your collection of single oils. With just a few versatile oils like Lavender, Frankincense, Peppermint, Lemon, and Patchouli, you can already address a wide range of magical intentions. As you desire to work with more specific energies, you can add single oils to your collection to meet those needs.

Blends or synergies are premixed combinations of essential oils formulated for specific purposes or intentions. Blends may be formulated to address certain specific wellness needs (e.g., a "breathe" blend, a "sweet dreams" blend, or a "tummy" blend), or they may be formulated to empower magical intentions (e.g., an "abundance" blend, a "joy" blend, or a "freedom" blend). Sometimes these blends are sold somewhat diluted (i.e., they contain carrier oil), and sometimes they are pure synergies that you can diffuse, use neat, or dilute yourself. If you have a specific intention you want to work toward, a premade blend from a source you trust is a more economical option in the short term. Some of my favorite and most effective oil blends contain a combination of oils that would be quite costly to purchase individually all at once and mix myself. However, purchasing a blend or two to use in spellwork or add to my daily rituals is quite affordable.

Blends are not usually as versatile as a collection of single oils, but many blends are more multipurpose than they may seem at first glance. A blend formulated for abundance may contain oils that are also well suited for love and romance, for example, or one formulated for peace and relaxation may also be helpful to facilitate meditation and healing.

Personally, I would recommend starting with a few multipurpose single oils such as those mentioned earlier, or any from this book that you feel drawn to, and one or two intention-specific blends and building your oil apothecary from there. You can benefit from the magic of essential oils without owning every single one, and learning what oils can be substituted (see chapter 4) is a great way to start learning about their properties and how they work.

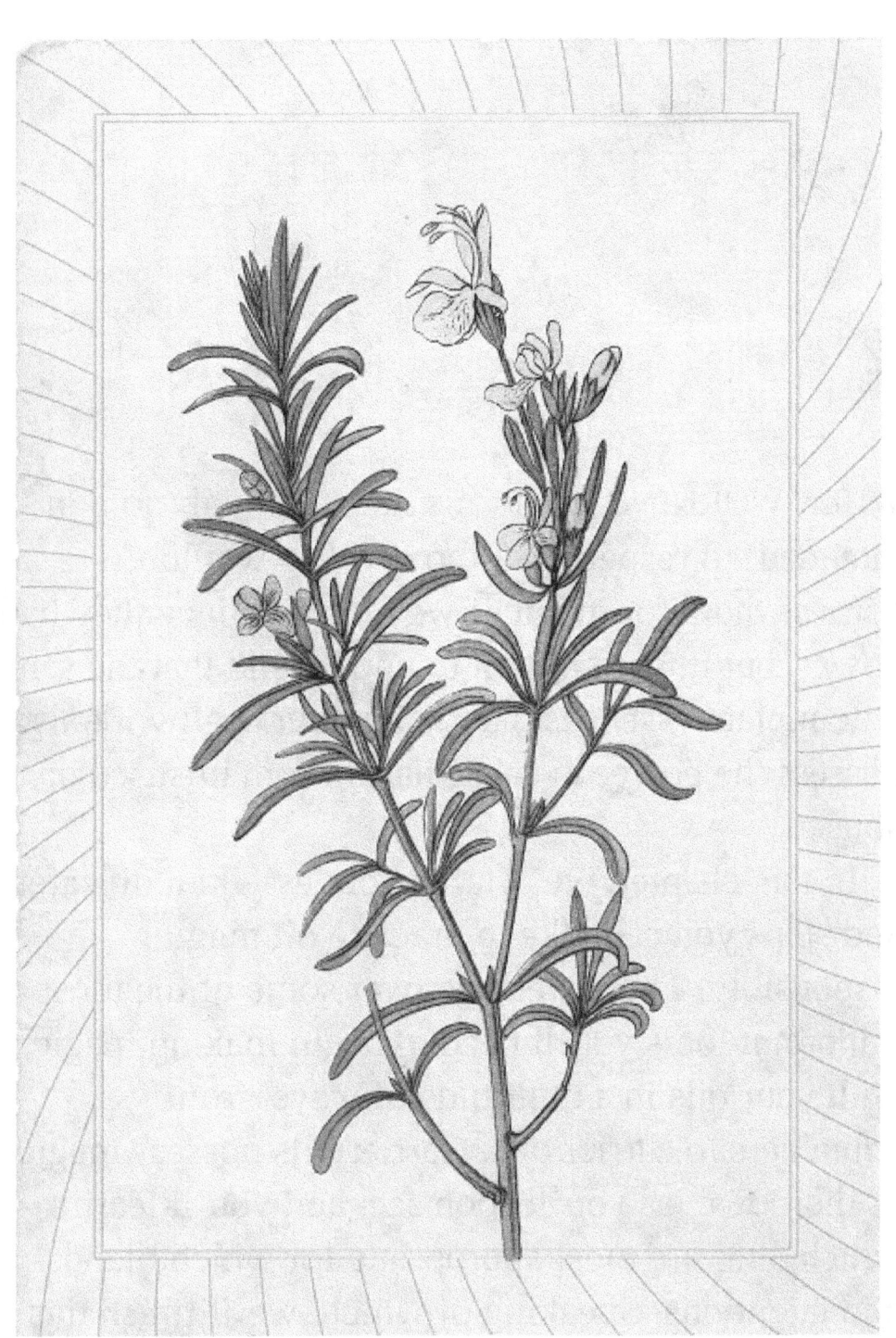

CHAPTER 4

Working with Oils

WHEN WORKING WITH oils, it's essential (no pun intended) to respect their power. We wouldn't harness them for magic if we didn't believe they had power, but it is important to understand that the same potent plant essences that bolster our spellwork also possess the power to cause harm when misused or abused.

In this chapter, we'll talk about essential oil safety and steps you can take to practice oil magic responsibly. Then, we'll go over some of the most important tools you'll need to begin making magic with your oils in a multitude of ways, from containers to carrier oils. Carrier oils possess magic of their own, as you'll soon see, and you'll learn which ones are most appropriate for which blends and intentions. Speaking of which, we'll finish this chapter by briefly discussing the arts of blending oils, crafting herbal-infused oils, and making substitutions.

Practicing Safety

It's easy to make the mistake of thinking that because something is natural it's completely safe. Lots of natural things, from mushrooms to mercury, can be quite harmful. Many more things that possess helpful and positive powers when used properly can cause harm when used irresponsibly or in excess. Essential oils are wonderful allies *when used responsibly*, but responsible usage requires research, care, and common sense.

We discussed the topic of neat usage in chapter 3, but for emphasis, I will repeat that if you are using an oil undiluted, only do so for a very good reason, and only if you have researched the particular oil or blend of oils you are using.

The first time you use an oil topically, patch test it to see if you have an existing sensitivity. To patch test, apply one or two drops of a diluted essential oil to a small clean spot on your inner forearm, and cover the spot with a bandage. If testing multiple oils simultaneously, separate them by a few inches and label the bandages with the name of each oil. Keep dry and covered for 24 hours unless you experience irritation in the area, in which case, remove the bandage and wash with soap and water. If an oil passes the patch test, you can confidently continue to use it on yourself topically. If not, find a substitute or leave it out of your blends.

Keep in mind also that oils affect every person differently. One of my best friends wears a blend containing Cinnamon Bark neat as a perfume (which I would personally *not* advise, but she herself has yet to experience any adverse reaction), whereas the first time I tried it, my entire forearm broke out in a burning rash. From her personal experience alone, my friend couldn't have known how that blend would affect me, because our skin and our sensitivities are not the same. As for me, I had *not* done my research, had no idea that Cinnamon Bark oil contains high levels of cinnamaldehyde, a known allergen, and should therefore typically be diluted to a maximum of

0.2 percent strength, and I did not yet know about sensitization. I am sharing what I've learned so that you don't *have* to learn the hard way.

Speaking of lessons you don't want to learn the hard way, most citrus oils and several other oils are phototoxic—that is, they cause photosensitivity when applied to the skin. Bitter Orange, Bergamot, Angelica, Cumin, Grapefruit, Lemon, Lime, and several other oils can cause severe burns when applied to skin that is then exposed to UV radiation (e.g., sunlight or tanning beds). In their book *Essential Oil Safety*, Robert Tisserand and Rodney Young recommend that if you use these oils topically, apply them somewhere that will not be exposed to sunlight for at least the next few days, or use approximately a 0.5 percent dilution rate.

If you are planning on using essential oils internally, to address any specific health concerns you may have or if you are taking blood-thinning medications or are pregnant or breastfeeding, it may be wise to consult with a certified aromatherapist. Notably, children and pets—especially cats—have specific needs concerning essential oils, so if you are planning to use oils on or around animals or children, a certified aromatherapist may be able to help guide you to make safe choices.

What You Need

To begin making magic out of your own home oil apothecary, you will need more than just essential oils. With oils and a diffuser, you can transform the energy of your sacred space, but if you want to put your plant magic to topical use, you'll need containers and carrier oils to make your own perfumes and potions. A selection of bottles, jars, and fatty oils will go a long way toward expanding the possibilities of your potion-making, but if you want to expand your practice even more, or simply make things easier on yourself, you may want a few additional tools and ingredients.

In this section, we'll go over some of the basic tools, containers, and carrier oils you might need. If you wish to complete all the spells in this book, a few other items to add to your home apothecary are noted in chapter 5 (see here).

Tools

No matter how you choose to incorporate essential oils into your magical practice and your daily life, you'll want to have these tools on hand. Some will help you smell the oils, and some will help you blend them, but all of them will help simplify and streamline the practice of oil magic.

Diffusers are a must. Ultrasonic diffusers are the most popular. They use distilled water and ultrasonic vibrations to disperse essential oils through the air in a pleasant mist. Passive diffusers use porous materials to absorb essential oils and slowly release their aromas. Some passive diffusers clip onto car vents or can be worn as diffuser jewelry. Cotton balls made of 100 percent cotton can be used as passive diffusers as well.

Nasal inhalers are ideal for on-the-go inhalation of favorite oils or custom blends. They're also perfect for inhaling oils for more than a few seconds, so you can keep your caps on your precious bottles.

Essential oil key tools are thin but sturdy pieces of metal, and sometimes plastic, used to remove and replace roller ball tops and orifice reducers. If you don't have one, you can use a thin knife, but you will risk damaging the piece you're trying to remove.

Pipettes are small disposable plastic droppers for transferring oils from one place to another. Some are graduated and labeled for measuring precise amounts.

Funnels in small and medium sizes are useful for pouring carrier oils into bottles with small openings. If your carrier oils have pump tops, you may not need these.

Containers

Essential oils and the things you make with them should always be stored in glass containers, as essential oils can degrade plastic over time, which in turn contaminates the oil. Amber glass is best to prevent sun damage, and blue glass is second best. Clear glass is okay if you intend to store the containers in a dark place, such as an opaque bag or box, or the refrigerator. Listed here are some of the most commonly used and trusted containers for essential oils.

Roller bottles are an absolute staple for oil magic. They are the easiest way to use oils topically and are perfect to keep with your self-care supplies, spellcasting tools, or to carry with you wherever you go. The most popular size is 10 milliliters, but 5-milliliter roller bottles are also available. You may also want to purchase a pouch or carrying case designed to keep a few bottles safe while on the go.

Spray bottles in 2-ounce and 4-ounce sizes are perfect for making room sprays and facial mists, and 16-ounce spray bottles are great for housing household cleansers with essential oils.

Mini bottles ranging from 1 to 5 milliliters with either orifice reducers or dropper tops are great for making your own synergies to be diluted later or diffused as is. They're also great for sharing samples with friends.

More bottles! Pretty perfume bottles are not necessary, but they can add some extra special magic to your anointing oils, candle dressing oils, and so on. Widemouthed jars are great for salves and for infusing your own carrier oils.

Carrier Oils

Carrier oils are fatty, nonvolatile oils that are used to dilute and "carry" essential oils. Because carrier oil molecules are heavier than essential oil molecules, they don't rise into the air as easily and, therefore, don't typically have much of an aroma. Some of them, like olive oil, coconut oil, and avocado oil, you may recognize from cooking. Others, like jojoba oil, rosehip seed oil, and argan oil, you may recognize from hair and skincare products.

You will need at least one good carrier oil in your apothecary to start working with essential oils safely. (If you do start with just one, I recommend jojoba.) I used fractionated coconut oil (FCO) as my sole carrier oil for months before I started experimenting with other carriers. Then, I tried jojoba oil and grapeseed oil, both of which I now prefer to FCO, as they are lighter and better for my skin. Finally, I started experimenting with other carrier oils, like rosehip seed oil, apricot kernel oil, and even camellia (tea) seed oil. Each of these has their own applications and benefits both practically and magically, and we'll dive into the specifics of a few preferred carriers later on in this chapter.

Dilution

As previously discussed, while there are times when it may be appropriate to use oils neat, most of the time you will want to dilute them to avoid skin irritation and sensitization. In addition to being generally safer, diluting your oils is also more economical. High-quality essential oils can be costly, but with proper dilution they can last for many uses. Suspending your essential oils in a carrier oil can also help you spread them more easily across larger areas of the body.

The bottles your essential oils come in should be labeled with suggested dilution instructions, but here are some general rules: Body care applications such as lotions, serums, and massage oils should contain about 2 percent essential oil; small-area topical applications such as roller bottles and perfumes can contain higher percentages (many experts suggest 5 percent); and hot oils such as Cinnamon, Clove, Thyme, and Oregano should be diluted to the lowest concentrations (less than 0.5 percent). Of course, your body chemistry and sensitivity may vary, so you may need to experiment to find what works for you. Typically, you want to use the lowest concentration that is effective for you.

Note that water is *not* a carrier oil. Oil and water do not mix. Diluting essential oils in water requires an emulsifier such as Castile soap, high-proof alcohol (Everclear or other 190-proof alcohol is best), or polysorbate 20.

Refer to the handy dilution chart on the next page. To use this chart, select the desired dilution percentage from the rows on the left and the desired amount of carrier oil from the columns at the top. Where that row and column meet, you will find the number of drops of essential oil needed to achieve approximately that dilution percentage in that amount of carrier oil. The values in this dilution chart are based on an assumption of 250 drops per 15 milliliters, rounding 1 fluid ounce to 30 milliliters (actually 29.57), and rounding to the nearest drop. Dilutions that would require significantly less than one drop are omitted and indicated with a (-).

Keep in mind that the suggested oil amounts are for the total amount of essential oils relative to the total amount of carrier. For this reason, you may sometimes want to create synergies, or blends of pure essential oils, to be used in multiple applications and add drops of the synergy to your carrier instead of adding each oil to the carrier individually.

		AMOUNT OF CARRIER OIL					
		5 ML	10 ML	15 ML	1 OZ	2 OZ	4 OZ
DILUTION PERCENTAGE	0.05%	-	-	-	-	-	1
	0.10%	-	-	-	-	1	2
	0.50%	-	1	1	3	5	10
	1%	1	2	3	5	10	20
	2%	2	3	5	10	20	40
	3%	3	5	8	15	30	60
	5%	4	8	13	25	50	100
	10%	8	17	25	50	100	200

Types of Carrier Oils

Just as every essential oil is different, every carrier oil is different. They have different viscosities, affect the skin in different ways, and possess different magical properties.

We say a carrier oil is "light" or "dry" when it feels thin and seeps into the skin quickly, or that it is "heavy" or "slow-drying" when it feels thicker and takes longer to soak into the skin. In general, lighter oils like jojoba tend to be noncomedogenic (i.e., they don't clog pores), whereas heavier oils such as coconut oil can be comedogenic. Everyone's skin is different, however, and will react uniquely to each oil, so if you're looking to start a magical skincare routine, you may need to experiment a bit to find the right oils for you.

In general, a carrier oil will possess the same magical properties as the plant it is derived from. For example, olive oil is associated with peace and protection, and avocado oil with love, beauty, and fertility. The magical properties and certain other characteristics of several common carrier oils are detailed here.

Coconut Oil

COCOS NUCIFERA

DESCRIPTION: Coconut oil is derived from the meat of the coconut and is sold in a few forms. Virgin coconut oil is solid at room temperature, whereas fractionated coconut oil (FCO) is liquid at room temperature, as it has had the long-chain triglycerides (lauric acid) removed. It is ruled by the Moon and the element of water. As carrier oils go, virgin and fractionated coconut oil are both very affordable, ranging from $0.20 to $2.00 an ounce at most retailers.

GOOD FOR: Coconut is associated with protection, fertility, health, abundance, and connection to the divine. As it is associated with the Moon, it is appropriate for all lunar magic and all the intentions that go with it. Practically, it nourishes skin and seals in moisture.

PROS AND CONS: Coconut oil is a very thick oil and can be drying to skin and hair but is good for use in massage. It is comedogenic and can clog pores. Virgin coconut oil possesses antimicrobial properties, but FCO does not. Both types of coconut oil are high in medium-chain triglycerides (MCTs). Because it is solid at room temperature, virgin coconut oil is not suitable for roller bottles and other liquid applications.

STORAGE: Store coconut oil (both types) in a cool, dark, and dry place. Refrigeration is not required but may extend the shelf life of the oil.

RECOMMENDATIONS: Solid coconut oil is recommended for Soothing Salve, and FCO would be a good choice for the moon-charged Auric Protection Pendant.

Olive Oil

OLEA EUROPAEA

DESCRIPTION: Olive oil is cold-pressed from olives, and while some olive oil is then refined and blended, extra-virgin olive oil (EVOO) is left pure and unrefined. For purposes of magic and self-care, you always want EVOO, as it will retain much more of the antioxidants and anti-inflammatories as well as the qi of the original olive tree. Olive is ruled by the Sun and the element of fire. Even organic EVOO can be purchased for less than $1 an ounce, making it very affordable. Be aware that olive oil is often adulterated with other lower quality oils, so be sure to purchase from a brand you trust if you want the real thing.

GOOD FOR: A favorite of Cleopatra and a symbol of Athena, olive oil is associated with peace, prosperity, healing, and the home. It is also associated with all things love and sex. Use it to bring peace and good fortune to relationships and the home, or to attract love or money. EVOO is great for dry and mature skin.

PROS AND CONS: Olive oil is thick and slow-drying, making it great for massage but not so good for acne-prone skin. While many people find the smell of olive oil to be quite pleasant, its aroma can overpower many essential oils.

STORAGE: Olive oil should be stored tightly sealed in a cool, dark place to preserve its shelf life. Once opened, high-quality EVOO should be used within a few months, but can last up to 18 months unopened.

RECOMMENDATIONS: If you don't mind the aroma, olive oil would be a good choice in Yummy Love Scrub, Lovers' Massage Oil, and Moontime Roller.

Jojoba Oil

SIMMONDSIA CHINENSIS

DESCRIPTION: What is known as jojoba "oil" is in fact a liquid wax extracted from the bean of the evergreen jojoba shrub native to the southwestern United States. It is a lightweight oil with a faint, nutty fragrance, is the most similar to sebum (the oil our bodies naturally produce), and can help calm and balance naturally oily skin. Jojoba is ruled by Jupiter and the element of fire. Good quality jojoba oil tends to run from $3 to $4 an ounce, making it pricier than coconut and olive oil, but well worth the cost for the love of your skin.

GOOD FOR: Jojoba is most commonly associated with perseverance, strength, and determination. Use it to invoke success and boost the power of your intentions, whatever they may be. Jojoba oil can also be used for purposes of purification, renewal, comfort, and healing. It is ideal for facial applications and anointing. Skin and hair alike love jojoba.

PROS AND CONS: Jojoba oil is lightweight and similar to your skin's natural oil (sebum), so it seeps into skin quickly, is noncomedogenic, and can be used to cleanse and unclog pores. It penetrates deep into the skin. Because it is a liquid wax, it has a very long shelf life.

STORAGE: True jojoba oil is shelf stable and does not oxidize or turn rancid. It can be stored indefinitely.

RECOMMENDATIONS: Jojoba oil would be a good choice for any spell, but especially preparations for the face and hair such as Third Eye Anointing Oil and Straw into Gold Hair Oil, and for prosperity potions like Liquid Gold Body Wash.

Grapeseed Oil

VITIS VINIFERA

DESCRIPTION: Grapeseed oil is a by-product of the wine industry and can therefore be obtained relatively cheaply ($0.50 to $2 an ounce depending on the source). It has a myriad of benefits, such as its reported abilities to boost collagen, lighten scars, smooth and firm skin, lessen redness, and even skin tone. It is a lightweight oil with no scent and is typically only available as a refined oil. Grapes are ruled by the Moon and the element of water.

GOOD FOR: Grapes have sometimes been known as the food of the gods, and grapeseed oil is suitable for all workings having to do with spirituality and divinity. It is also an appropriate ingredient for fertility spells and can be invoked to bring joy, ease introductions and smooth relationships, foster growth, and increase abundance and prosperity. Grapeseed oil is nourishing and healing to the skin, and suitable for even the most sensitive skin types.

PROS AND CONS: Because grapeseed oil is so lightweight, it is great for all types of skin and is absorbed quickly. It is touted for a plethora of skin benefits and has little to no smell, so it will not interfere with the aroma of essential oils. However, it does have a shorter shelf life than other oils.

STORAGE: Store in a cool, dark place and use within three to six months. Kept refrigerated, grapeseed oil can last up to a year.

RECOMMENDATIONS: Grapeseed oil would be an ideal carrier oil for Intuition Roller, Soothsayer's Soak, or Let the Good Times Roll.

Avocado Oil
PERSEA AMERICANA

DESCRIPTION: Avocado oil is produced from the avocado fruit, which is native to Mexico. It is a heavier oil and is purported to be good for dry, mature, and sun-damaged skin. It is also used in cooking and has a relatively high smoke point. It is ruled by Venus and the element of water. Cosmetic-grade avocado oil tends to run between $1 and $2 an ounce, making it very affordable.

GOOD FOR: Avocados are associated with virility, fertility, love, lust, beauty, wealth, and abundance. Avocado oil is also associated with wellness and healing. The fruit and the oil are both sensual and luxurious. Avocado oil is an ideal carrier oil for topical love potions of all kinds, romantic massage oils, beauty-enhancing masks, and all kinds of oil magic for manifesting abundance.

PROS AND CONS: Avocado oil is a heavier oil but is relatively noncomedogenic, so it is usually suitable even for sensitive, oily, or acne-prone skin. It is thick and slow-drying enough to make a great massage oil and has little to no aroma of its own.

STORAGE: Store avocado oil in a cool, dark place, or in the refrigerator to extend its shelf life from 6–8 months to 9–12 months.

RECOMMENDATIONS: Avocado oil would be perfect in Lovers' Massage Oil, Love Potion No. 10, or Good Fortune Fizz.

Sweet Almond Oil
PRUNUS DULCIS

DESCRIPTION: Sweet almond oil is pressed from ripe almonds and can be purchased refined or unrefined (for magical and skincare purposes, you want unrefined). A favorite of aromatherapists and skincare enthusiasts, sweet almond oil is a lightweight carrier oil touted for its skin-healing properties. It is ruled by Mercury and the element of air. Unrefined sweet almond oil generally runs from $1.50 to $3 an ounce.

GOOD FOR: Almonds are associated with money, prosperity, wisdom, and sobriety, and sweet almond oil is associated with sweetness (of course), innocence, protection, purification, and true love. Use sweet almond oil as a base in oil magic for any of these purposes.

PROS AND CONS: Although it is unsuitable for anyone with a tree nut allergy, sweet almond oil is nourishing, healing, and suitable for most skin types. It is a dry oil that seeps into skin quickly. It stores well in most conditions but has a maximum shelf life of about one year unopened, or six months once opened.

SAFETY CONSIDERATIONS: Anyone with a tree nut allergy should not use sweet almond oil or other nut oils.

STORAGE: Keep tightly sealed and away from extreme heat.

RECOMMENDATIONS: Sweet almond oil would be perfect as a base in Yummy Love Scrub, Aphrodite's Bath, or Straw into Gold Hair Oil.

Apricot Kernel Oil
PRUNUS ARMENIACA

DESCRIPTION: Apricot kernel oil is pressed from the kernels found in the centers of apricot pits. It is a nourishing, lightweight oil and is easily absorbed by the skin. It is similar to sweet almond oil and is popular as an alternative to sweet almond oil for people with nut allergies. Apricot is ruled by Venus and the element of water. Quality apricot kernel oil runs from about $1.50 to $3 an ounce, about the same as sweet almond oil.

GOOD FOR: Apricots and apricot kernel oil are associated with sweetness, love, beauty, peace, and protection. They are also tied to female fertility, the divine feminine, and protection of women. Additionally, apricot kernel oil is appropriate in magic focused on creativity, longevity, and balance.

PROS AND CONS: Apricot kernel oil is more costly than some other oils, but it is also more nourishing and healing for the skin than many other carrier oils. It has a longer shelf life than its cousin sweet almond oil.

SAFETY CONSIDERATIONS: Although skin contact reactions are rare, it's always a good idea to patch test before use.

STORAGE: Store in a cool, dark place for up to one year.

RECOMMENDATIONS: Consider using apricot kernel oil in Moontime Roller, Goddess Body Wash, or Roll-On Energy Shield.

Rosehip Seed Oil

ROSA CANINA, ROSA RUBIGINOSA

DESCRIPTION: Rosehip seed oil is pressed from the small hairy seeds found inside rosehips, the fruits of wild rose bushes. It takes a vast amount of rosehip seeds to produce a small amount of oil, and the itchy hairs must be carefully strained from the finished product. All this explains why rosehip seed oil is one of the more costly carrier oils, coming in at around $5 to $10 an ounce from most retailers. It is ruled by Venus and the element of water.

GOOD FOR: Extremely nourishing to skin and especially good for the face, rosehip seed oil can be used anytime you want to call upon the magic of rose. Inseparable from the divine feminine and sacred to many goddesses, rose is associated with love, romance, and sexuality; fertility, abundance, and manifestation; and protection, peace, and emotional healing. Use rosehip seed oil in workings for any of these intentions.

PROS AND CONS: Rosehip seed oil has significant anti-inflammatory and antioxidant properties but must be used within a few months of opening. It is also quite costly among carrier oils.

STORAGE: Rosehip seed oil has a shelf life of about six months when stored well-sealed in a cool, dark, and dry place. Refrigerate this oil to maximize its shelf life.

RECOMMENDATIONS: Rosehip seed oil would be ideal for Auric Protection Pendant, Aphrodite's Bath, or Love Potion No. 10.

More Carrier Oils

There are many more carrier oils available than those listed in the previous section. Here are a few others you may wish to include in your oil magic:

Argan oil is a luxurious tree nut oil from Morocco that is popular for conditioning hair and skin. Sometimes called "liquid gold," it could be used in magic for prosperity, abundance, love, and beauty.

Camellia seed oil (from the tea plant *Camellia sinensis*, not "tea tree" *Melaleuca alternifolia*) is lightweight and silky, and can be used to incorporate the gentle, gracious, loving, and healing qi of tea into oil magic.

Castor oil is often used to support healthy hair growth and skin healing. Magically, it can be used for protection and healing.

Evening primrose oil is associated with the Moon and women's wellness. It is appropriate for divination, lunar magic, and assisting with balance, cycles, and feminine healing.

Moringa oil is pressed from the seeds of the moringa tree, which some call the tree of life, and has a history of medicinal and cosmetic use dating back to ancient Egypt. It is ideal for manifestation magic.

Pomegranate seed oil is associated with divine knowledge, the underworld, wisdom, and blood mysteries. Use it in divination magic.

Blending

You can blend oils to combine the magic of multiple botanicals into one intentional potion. When you blend together multiple oils with similar magical properties, they multiply and magnify each other's qi. When you blend oils that have different magical properties, they can help narrow down your intention to be more specific. For example, Black Pepper and Clove are both protective, so blending them together would amplify their protective powers, whereas Clary Sage helps open the third eye and Rose is associated with love, so a blend of Clary Sage and Rose could encourage visions related to love and relationships or strengthen intuition with regard to romance and potential partners.

Working with a particular blend also allows your brain to store that blend's unique scent in its library of scent memories along with whatever associations you program the memory with. For example, you may already have several memories associated with rosemary, but the unique smell of blended Rosemary, Lavender, and Patchouli may have no associations for you yet. You can make that blend with a specific intention in mind and specific affirmations on your tongue, and work with it repeatedly using that intention and affirmation to create a new olfactory memory. From then on, working with that blend may help you tune in to that intention even subconsciously. In psychological terms, this is called context-dependent memory. For example, I have a blend I work with specifically to help me get out of bed in the morning with energy and purpose, and another blend I use specifically for money magic and strengthening my abundance mindset.

This book contains a plethora of suggestions for magical oil blends and how to use them, but you can also learn to create and use your own blends. When blending oils for magic, there are three basic factors you want to keep in mind.

First, know the physical and chemical properties of the oils you intend to use and any safety considerations. Are any of them hot oils? If you intend to use your blend topically, are any of the oils phototoxic? Are they safe to use while pregnant or breastfeeding?

Second, know the magical properties of the oils you want to blend. This book contains complete profiles of 30 of my most-used magical oils, which should be plenty to get you started. Knowing the magical properties of your oils will help you select oils that match your intention and enhance each other's energetic actions.

Third, the aromas of the oils you combine should complement one another to create a pleasing finished product. After all, if you don't enjoy the smell of a blend, you probably won't want to work with it. The oil profiles in chapter 6 include suggestions for blending, but your nose is your best guide. The nose knows! When I'm planning a blend, I like to line up the oils I'm considering, remove their lids, and smell the opened bottles all together. If that combined scent feels good, I'll start building the blend drop by drop in a 2- or 3-milliliter bottle, keeping a written tally of how many drops of each I add. When I'm happy with the aroma, I write down the finished recipe and my intention for the blend so that I can replicate it later.

Infused Oils

WHEREAS ESSENTIAL OILS are the lightweight aromatic compounds or essence of a plant extracted through distillation, infused oils are carrier oils that have soaked up some of the properties and fat-soluble compounds, including essential oils as well as heavier fatty oils, of other herbs via infusion. The process is a lot like making a tea or tisane, but with oil instead of water, less heat, and more time.

You can use any carrier oil you like (I prefer to make large batches using oils with a longer shelf life) and any nontoxic herbs you desire. I love infusing locally foraged finds into jojoba or FCO, such as the ash juniper that grows all over central Texas. Just be certain you know the identity of the plants you infuse and their properties. Infusing carrier oils is a great way to incorporate the energies of plants you have in dried form but may not have access to in essential oil form. Some of my favorite plants to infuse are St. John's wort, calendula, chrysanthemum, rose, and, of course, vervain. (See the Resources section at the end of this book for recommended reading on herbalism and herbal magic to inspire your own choices.)

My chosen method for making herbal-infused oils is slow and does not involve heat. For this method, choose a decently widemouthed glass jar, sterilize it by boiling or with high-proof alcohol, and then let it air-dry. Wearing sterile gloves, fill the jar with completely dry plant matter (you *can* use fresh, but there is a risk that the moisture will cause mold to grow in your oil), leaving an inch or two of room at the top. Pour your carrier oil of choice into the jar, completely covering the plant matter (exposed plant matter also poses a mold risk).

At this stage, I like to add one or more substantial crystals, both to help weigh down the plant matter so it stays submerged as well as to infuse the oil with intention. If you do this, be sure to only use crystals that are safe for direct infusion. (To be considered safe for use, a crystal must have a Mohs' scale hardness of 6 or greater and must not contain toxic minerals that could leach into the oil. Rose quartz, citrine, amethyst, clear quartz, obsidian, and aventurine are good options for a variety of intentions.) You may choose to inscribe your jar with sigils, runes, affirmations, or another type of written spell. You may also choose to affix images that represent intentions you would like to imbue into the oil. Feel free to keep it simple and skip the woo-woo stuff altogether, or to make the magic as complex as you like. You can chant into your oil, tie it with colored ribbon representing your intentions, or even build a crystal grid around the jar wherever you decide to store it.

Store the jar in a cool, dark place for one full moon cycle (i.e., one month), checking it every so often to be sure the plant matter stays submerged. You may want to agitate the jar periodically, but this is optional. When the infusion is complete, strain out the solids with cheesecloth and transfer to a sterile glass container for storage. (I like to keep mine in dropper bottles or pump bottles for ease of use.) Store your infused oil the same way you would store the carrier oil it is made from. You can use infused oils as a base for roller bottles, massage oil, bath oil (add to the bath alone, with Epsom salt, or as part of bath bombs), or any other way you would use a carrier oil.

Substitution

As you start your journey down the oily side of the plant-magic path and build your personal oil apothecary, there will be occasions when you will want to do a spell or create a blend that calls for an oil you don't yet have. When this happens, you'll be glad to know you can often substitute one oil for another!

The principles of substitution vary based on your reason for working with an oil. Most sources suggest substitutions based on chemical constituents and physical effects of an oil, as most resources on essential oils are focused on using them for health and wellness. This is totally valid, and if you intend to use your oils in that way, you will want to adhere to that principle and follow those suggestions. Other sources suggest substitutions based on fragrance notes and substituting an oil with another oil that has a similar aroma, because their goal is to create a particular aroma. That said, the substitutions I suggest throughout chapter 6 and in the Substitutions Chart are based primarily on magical intention.

When deciding on a replacement for a missing oil, first refer to the list of suggested substitutions and see if any stand out to you. Then read up on the individual oils suggested to make sure the one you want to use shares the specific properties you require. For example, you may substitute Eucalyptus for Chamomile in energy cleansing situations, but probably not for sleep support.

In oil magic, what is most important when selecting and substituting oils is your intention and how the plant essences harmonize energetically with your goals. The therapeutic effects and aroma may—and ideally should—complement the magical effects, but when it comes down to it, they are secondary to the qi and any personal associations you may have.

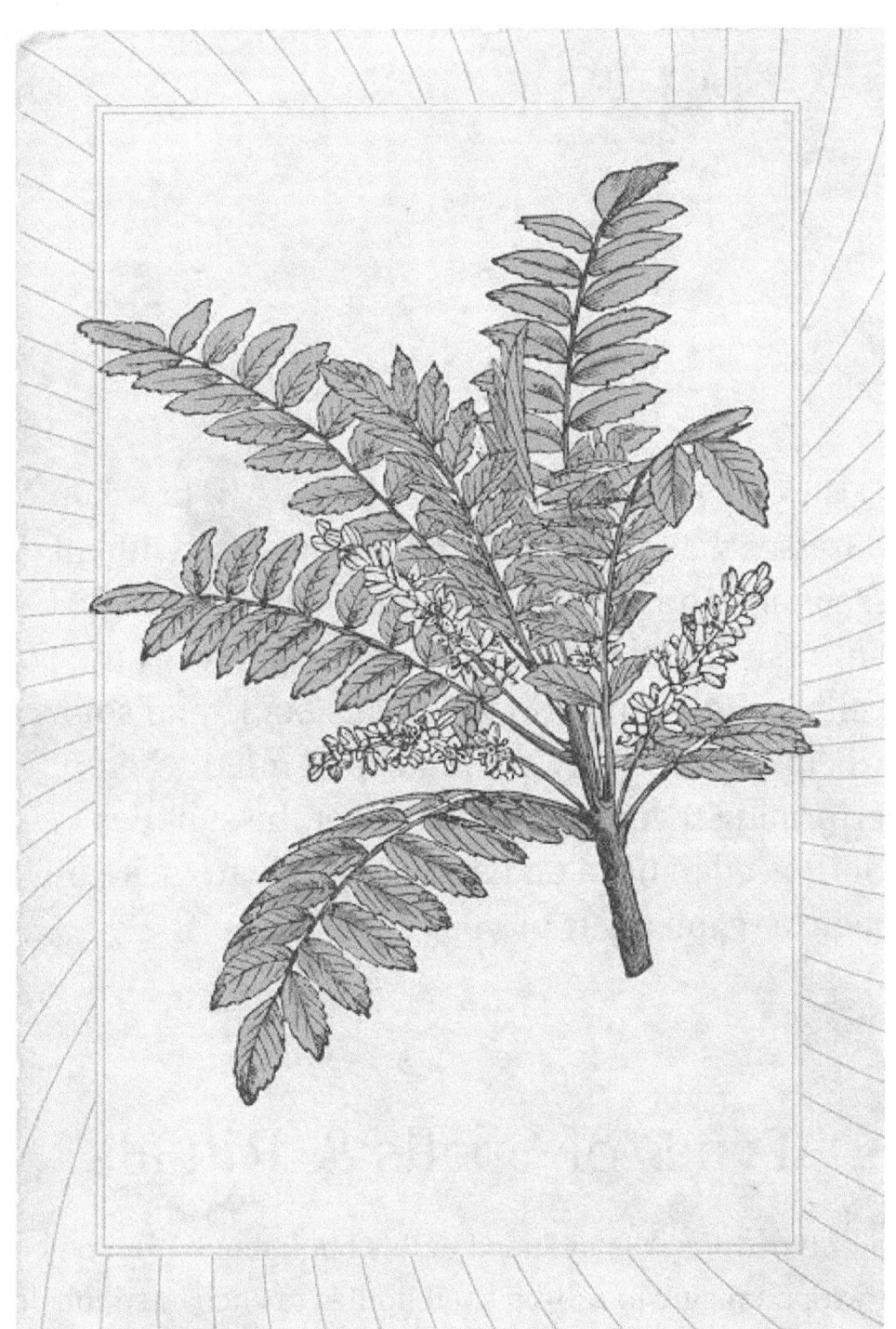

CHAPTER 5

Practicing Magic

SO HOW DO you actually *do* oil magic? This chapter addresses that question in a general sense with all the essential information you need to practice magic. We'll talk about the 12 different major types of spells included in part four of this book, and some principles you may want to keep in mind when performing them. We'll also cover the supplies you'll need to have on hand to be able to make oil magic a regular part of your craft.

Types of Spells & Rituals

The 12 major types of spells included in this book range from objects enchanted with oil magic to roll-on spell bottles to enchanted inhalers to personal care potions infused with various intentions. Read on to learn all about them! Use this chapter as a guide to the spells in this book, and as a jumping-off point for crafting your own spells.

Charms, Talismans & Enchanted Objects

Because essential oils have such potent magical energy and their aromas can stimulate our minds and memories in such powerful and particular ways, they can be used to charm, enchant, or otherwise charge magical objects with intention. This can be as simple as charging a crystal with a few drops of a blended synergy (Pocket Pyrite) or as complex as creating your own salt dough rune set infused with oily plant magic (Rose Runes). This book includes suggestions for charmed jewelry (Auric Protection Pendant; Freyja's Necklace), enchanted journals (Gratitude Journal; Divination Journal), charm bags (Four Corners Fortification), and more.

Feel free to stray from the instructions in this book, if needed, in order to adapt the included enchantments or create your own from scratch, but when choosing where to apply your oils, keep in mind that essential oils can break down many plastics and paints.

As with most magic, affirmations or incantations and visualizations (visual, emotional, and somatic) help infuse and affirm your intentions for your magical objects and can be repeated along with a reapplication of oils to refresh and recharge the enchantment.

Enchanted Roller Bottles

Roller bottles are the perfect portable potions. Small enough to pop in a bag or a pocket, they can still pack a magical punch, and they make applying oils on the go easy and mess-free. The bottles themselves come in several sizes, although 10 milliliters is considered the standard, and are fitted with a roller ball top that allows easy application to the skin. You can make rollers for just about anything, and the enchanted roller bottles in this book run the gamut from a topical potion for protection (Roll-On Energy Shield) to one for strengthening an abundance mindset (Let the Good Times Roll).

Generally, when making a roller bottle, you'll want to add the essential oils and let them mix (preferably for some time, though waiting is not absolutely necessary) to create a synergy before topping with carrier oil.

Roller bottles are the spell bottles of oil magic, but they don't act merely as a charm; you can use them continuously to reap the benefits of the enchantments bestowed upon them and the oils contained therein. As with spell bottles, you can add dried flowers and herbs or insoluble and nontoxic crystals (such as those suggested in the spells in this book) to your roller bottle creations, and the outside of your enchanted roller bottles can be decorated with appropriate runes, sigils, words, affirmations, or symbols if you desire.

Diffuser Spells

Diffuser spells can be done anywhere you can plug in a diffuser. Since diffusers spread, or "diffuse," oils throughout a living space, they are ideal for infusing a space in your home with a particular intention. You can set the mood for romance (In the Mood for Love), purify and protect your home (Clear the Air), attune a room to the energy of abundance (Make It Rain), or create an ideal space for divinatory work (Aura of Extrasensory Perception).

Most diffusers use ultrasonic vibration and distilled water to disperse oils. Using distilled water will prolong the diffuser's life by preventing mineral buildup, so I don't recommend using water collected from rain, snow, or elsewhere in nature, but you can totally make moon water with distilled water! Be sure to always clean your diffuser when switching magical intentions or as recommended by the manufacturer.

Note that this book includes recipes designed for 180-milliliter diffusers, so you can adjust the amounts up or down depending on your diffuser capacity or desired potency. If you wish to use one of the blends frequently, you may want to make and charge a "diffuser bomb": a small bottle of pre-blended oils that you can drop into a diffuser at a moment's notice. To make a diffuser bomb, multiply the recipe by the desired number of batches and swirl together in a small bottle with a dropper top or orifice reducer.

Spell Sprays

Spell sprays are a more portable version of diffuser spells. They allow you to spray yourself and your belongings, or even fill a physical space, with enchanting aromas. The spell sprays in this book are for such things as encouraging the wealth you put out into the world to return to you in abundance (Minting Money), inviting prophetic dreams (Prophetic Dreams Pillow Spray), and cleansing and hallowing the energy of a space (Sacred Space Spray).

The sprays in this book are water-based, but oil (including essential oils) and water do not mix, so emulsifiers must be used for the sprays to mix properly. The best emulsifiers for this purpose (and those suggested in chapters 7 to 11) are polysorbate 20 and alcohol. Polysorbate 20 should be used at a ratio of approximately one part polysorbate 20 to one part essential oils. If you use alcohol, Everclear or another 190-proof alcohol is best. The lower the alcohol content, the less effective it is. I do not recommend isopropyl (rubbing) alcohol, as the smell can overpower and conflict with the essential oils. High-proof alcohol, when used as an emulsifier, should be included as approximately 25 percent of the total solution volume, or more if the proof is lower.

Intentional Inhalers

Intentional breathing spells are the simplest to prepare and can be done anywhere at a moment's notice. They involve deeply inhaling oils while visualizing and may also include an affirmation or incantation.

The simple breath spells in this book (e.g., Inner Peace Inhaler; Get Intuit Anywhere) are written for use with aromatherapy inhalers. These "inhalers" are really just metal capsules (do not use plastic ones) that contain vented glass bottles filled with cotton wicks. You add a few drops of oil to the wick, and whenever you need its magic, you just open the capsule and inhale. I recommend purchasing a set of several different colors to have on hand for different oil blends and intentions.

If you don't have an inhaler, and you are only using very gentle oils, you may use the scent tent method, which involves applying a drop of essential oil directly to your palms and inhaling from your cupped hands. Scent tents are appropriate for infrequent use as long as none of the oils you are using are hot oils or known irritants. You could also apply your oils to a cotton ball made of 100 percent cotton and inhale from there.

Enchanted Oils

Technically, many things mentioned in this book could qualify as "enchanted oils," but here I am specifically addressing hair and body oils, massage oils, anointing oils, candle dressing oils, and the like. While you could place these oils in roller bottles, I personally prefer to keep them in dropper bottles, pump bottles, or in the case of anointing oils, perfume bottles with a glass dipping wand, and suggest that you might do the same.

This book includes instructions for enchanted oils intended to inspire passion between lovers (Lovers' Massage Oil), comfort sore muscles (Miracle Massage Oil), and enhance the luster of your locks while emanating an aura of abundance (Straw into Gold Hair Oil). These spells are very simple, and though the magic is enhanced with suggested affirmations and visualizations, the practical process is extremely straightforward: Just combine essential oils and add carrier oil. Ideally, you will allow the essential oils to sit together for some time—perhaps overnight—before adding carrier oil, but the waiting time is not absolutely necessary. Then, your enchanted oils are ready to use immediately.

Magical Bathing

Magical bathing is a wonderful way to cleanse your current energy and soak up the energy you desire. In the following chapters, you'll find spells to infuse your bathwater with an assortment of intentions from love (Aphrodite's Bath) and healing (Soothing Soak) to luck and prosperity (Good Fortune Fizz).

There are many ways to incorporate oil magic into your bath time, but they are not all equally effective. One option is to dilute essential oils with carrier oil and add them to bathwater, which makes for a pleasant and skin-nourishing experience but leaves the bath slippery and hard to clean. Some people merely add essential oils to Epsom salt, but this does not dilute the oils. Another option is to make a bubble bath by adding essential oils to one part distilled water, one part FCO, and two parts Castile soap. This makes for a fun and magical bath, and the soap fully emulsifies the oils into the water.

My favorite method of magical bathing is with homemade bath bombs. The fizzing action feels fun and magical, and once dissolved, the oils are fully emulsified in the bathwater, which becomes soothing and moisturizing to the skin. The base recipe used in this book can be adjusted to any intention by switching out the essential oils, but if you choose to get creative, be sure to avoid hot oils, as bathwater will come into contact with all of your most sensitive skin.

Blessed Body Washes

Homemade body washes for the shower make for the perfect prelude to a magical bath, or you can substitute them when a bath would be impossible or inconvenient. My favorite base recipe includes equal parts honey, carrier oil, and Castile soap, plus essential oils of choice. Not only does this body wash leave skin smooth, soft, and clean, but it also serves as an ideal vehicle for infusing the skin with the magic of your chosen oils. Plus, honey adds some versatile magic of its own.

Body wash spells, like many of the spells in this book, are often paired with affirmations or visualizations that add to their effectiveness. This book includes blessed body washes for self-love and sensuality (Goddess Body Wash), emotional healing (Wash Your Worries Away), and infusing your body with the energy of abundance (Liquid Gold Body Wash). Make one of these spells part of your daily routine or mix up a body wash with your signature scent and pair it with an affirmation of your choice to help yourself feel (and smell) amazing in your body every day.

Scrub Spells

Shower scrubs and body polishes allow you to exfoliate your skin while infusing it with plant magic in the form of oils. At their simplest, scrubs contain an exfoliating agent (usually sugar or salt, but the options are endless) and a carrier oil. Essential oils add plant magic and enchanting aromas, and I prefer to add Castile soap to avoid slippery shower syndrome and leave the skin feeling fresh and clean. For the scrubbing element, brown sugar is a very gentle exfoliant, white sugar is coarser, and salt is even coarser. Other exfoliants you can use include ground coffee, poppy seeds, baking soda, ground oatmeal, and powdered herbs.

In this book, you'll find scrub spells for protecting your energy (Protection Polish) and encouraging love and romance (Yummy Love Scrub). The recipes given can be adapted to any intention by switching out the essential oils accordingly, or you can experiment with other exfoliants. Just remember not to exfoliate too often, and to be gentle with your more sensitive skin. Scrubs must be stored in a dry place and must not be contaminated with moisture, to preserve their shelf life.

Balms & Salves

Balms and salves are oily blessings in solid form, thanks to a little help from beeswax. Balms tend to be more solid and have a higher beeswax content, such as the heart chakra balm (Anahata Opening) in chapter 8, whereas salves are less firm and have a lower beeswax content (e.g., Soothing Salve). The balm recipe in chapter 8 could be adapted with different essential oils to serve as a lip balm (try Lavender and Orange) or a solid perfume by adapting the oil blend from Third Eye Anointing Oil here. The salve recipe from chapter 9 could be similarly adapted by using the oil blends from Miracle Massage Oil, Love Potion No. 10, or Happy Tummy Roller. Additionally, balms and salves are especially good opportunities to use herbal-infused carrier oils, should you have any around.

Candle Magic

At first glance, it might seem that candle magic and oil magic are two wholly separate disciplines, but candle magic has long made use of magical oils for candle dressing. Candle dressing is the term used to describe the process of coating spell candles in enchanted oils appropriate to the purpose of the spell. The oils lend their magic to the candle spell, and as the candle burns, the oils are warmed and release their aromas and their qi. Should you choose to carve your candle first, dressing it with oils is also a way of consecrating and giving lifeblood to the carved words or symbols (similar to staining runes). In this book, you'll find candle spells for love (Like a Moth to a Flame) and divination (Inner Eye Illumination), but you can create your own candle dressing oil blends for any intention you can dream of.

I recommend candles made of 100 percent beeswax, both because they are all-natural and nontoxic and because of their long history of use in magic. They have a pleasant and mild scent and are associated with health, wealth, harmony, sweetness, love, and manifestation. If you're feeling inspired, you can even make your own beeswax candles and scent them with oils from within.

Bewitching Body Butters

Body butters are similar to balms, but instead of beeswax, their texture comes from natural butters such as shea butter, cocoa butter, or mango butter mixed in with the oils. Body butters are typically whipped, which lends them a luxurious texture and makes them easy to apply. They melt into the skin on contact and feel intensely nourishing, creating a protective coating that seals in both moisture and magical intention.

There is only one body butter recipe in this book (Midas Touch Body Butter), but it can be adapted to any magical goal by switching out the essential oils for oils that correspond to your intention. Consider making body butters with the essential oil blends from Protection Polish, Aphrodite's Bath, or Inner Peace Inhaler. The grapeseed oil can be switched for jojoba or another carrier, and shea butter is largely interchangeable with mango butter and cocoa butter, except that cocoa butter has a strong chocolate smell—a smell most find utterly delectable but tends to overpower the aroma of essential oils.

Charging & Enchantment

Often when we think of charging magical items, we think merely of setting them out in the moonlight or otherwise allowing them to "soak up" subtle energy from something else, such as a crystal—similar to plugging in your phone to charge. While charging *can* be as simple as this, it is much more effective when combined with the action of telling your magical items what to do—in other words, giving them a charge, *charging* them with the responsibility of a given task.

You can certainly charge your oils like this, and I often do. In truth, you are not only telling your oils what to do, but you are also—and possibly more importantly—communicating from your conscious to your subconscious mind and telling *yourself* what your charged oils are for. In other words, you are telling your body and mind what to do with the oil when you inhale it or absorb it through your skin. I like to combine this method of charging with the better-known method of moonlight-charging.

Each full moon, I gather a few essential oils and bring them outside or to a window. There, I say hello to the moon and start by expressing my gratitude for her light and all that has come to pass this month. Then I go through my oils one by one, giving each a charge or enchantment, taking a moment to visualize or attune to the charge or the oil, and then I inhale the oil deeply, cap it, and move on to the next. For example, during a recent full moon, I held up my bottle of Peppermint to the moon and said, "Peppermint, full of life, may you grant me energy, focus, motivation, and perseverance to do the things I know need to be done, so that I may be of better service to this world and everyone in it. This is your charge." Then I inhaled the Peppermint and tuned into the feelings of energy, focus, motivation, and perseverance for a few deep breaths, capped the bottle, and set it in the moonlight to charge overnight. In the morning, I said thank you to the moon and to every oil I charged that night. Then, I integrated those oils into my collection to be used and mixed into appropriate potions. You can do a similar charging ritual with a crystal or crystal grid with appropriate correspondences if the moon is not available, or you can combine crystal-charging and moonlight-charging into one ritual.

You may choose to do a ritual like this each time you acquire a new bottle of oil to direct and amplify its natural powers. Think how much more powerful the calming body wash (Wash Your Worries Away) would be if you had previously charged your Lavender with gently soothing the body, heart, and mind; Frankincense with opening the mind to new ideas and perspectives; and Orange with brightening and uplifting the mood. These charges are all aligned with the oils' natural magical properties, but charging with intention and purpose enhances and empowers the effects. If you're not sure what sort of charge to give an oil, refer to the oil profiles in chapter 6 and spend some time attuning to the energy of the oil.

Attunement

Attunement is the other side of charging or enchanting for working with essential oils. Because high-quality essential oils carry such strong qi naturally without any additional enchantment at all, often you can benefit from attuning yourself to the subtle energy of an oil rather than, or in addition to, charging it with additional enchantments.

One of the cool things about working with oils in this way is that when we inhale them or apply them topically, they permeate us with more than their subtle energy. Their actual chemical makeup permeates our cells and begins moving through our bodies. The simplest way to attune to the energy of an oil is simply to apply it, diluted, to your inner wrists and the back of your neck, and then inhale it deeply, either from the bottle, your hands, a cotton ball or diffuser, or an inhaler. Breathe deeply and notice how you feel in your heart, body, and mind as the oil enters your bloodstream. If you have researched an oil's magical and energetic properties, you may have some idea of what effect it might have. Do you find your experience matches your expectations, or are you experiencing something different?

After you have attuned to the energy of an oil once and can recognize that feeling in your heart, body, and mind, it will likelier be much easier to repeat the process in the future. Plus, you will now have an experiential understanding of the oil's effects on you and will be better able to concoct custom blends with the oils in your collection, having a deeper understanding of each oil.

For oils that you have already charged as described here or enchanted as in most of the spells in this book, when you attune to them, you are attuning not only to the natural qi of the oil but also to the enchantment or charge you placed upon them. In fact, most of the spells in this book are in two or three parts: First, the practical mixing of ingredients; second, the charging or enchanting of the product with visualizations and affirmations; and third, attuning to the product with each use. For example, you assemble a roller bottle, enchant it with your intention through visualization and affirmation, and then attune to the energy of the completed roller (oils, enchantment, and all) each time you repeat the affirmation and roll on the oils.

The Green Witch's Kitchen

The kitchen is the hearth and heart of the home and is the modern apothecary. Unless you are lucky enough to have a separate apothecary for potion-making in your home, you will probably concoct most of your oil magic in the kitchen, although you can *use* it just about anywhere. In this section, we'll cover what you'll need or want to have on hand in your kitchen or home apothecary to perform all the spells in this book.

Oils

You can't do oil magic without essential oils—they're essential! While you don't need a ton of them, the more you have in your collection, the more you can do with them. As long as you store them properly, you don't really need to worry about them going bad. So although there's no need to go hog wild, it's okay to stock up, and there are some essential oils you'll never want to run out of. Every oil witch will have a different list of must-haves, but the 30 oils detailed in chapter 6 are a good start to a solid collection. For the times when you *do* run out of a given oil, check the Substitutions Chart.

You'll also need carrier oils. A variety of options are detailed in chapter 4 (see here). Unlike essential oils, these can tend to go bad, so you don't want to buy more than you can use within an oil's shelf life. The exception to this is jojoba oil, which I personally buy in bulk since it does not deteriorate over time, and is one of my favorite carrier oils for topical use regardless.

Vitamin E oil is an optional addition to oil magic recipes. It can help prevent oxidation, so it can extend the shelf life of your oily concoctions and is good for skin, too. You only need a few drops—1 percent of the final product whenever you use it.

Other Ingredients

Besides oils, you'll need a few other ingredients to complete all the spells in this book. From shower scrubs and body washes to spell sprays and solid perfumes, here's an overview of what you'll need:

Castile soap: A necessary ingredient for body washes and shower scrubs, Castile soap is a top-notch emulsifier. You can also use it to make bubble baths, hand soap, and more.

Polysorbate 20: A very good emulsifier for combining essential oils and water, polysorbate 20 is used in all the spray recipes in this book. As detailed in the recipes, Everclear or another 190-proof alcohol can be used instead, if desired.

Beeswax: When you need to create something with a firmer texture, such as a balm or a solid perfume, beeswax is the way to go. It has a mild honey smell and also makes some of the best spell candles.

Honey: With its golden color and natural sweetness, honey is a perfect ingredient in love and prosperity spells. It's also a humectant, which means it adds moisture to skin.

Salt: A popular ingredient in protection spells, salt is also a natural exfoliant and dispersant. Use it in charm bags, shower scrubs, and more.

Sugar: With magical properties similar to honey, and skincare properties similar to salt, sugar is a gentle and effective exfoliant for use in shower scrubs.

Bath bomb ingredients: You'll only need these ingredients for making bath bombs, though after you've made them once, you'll want to do it again and again. The standard recipe I've provided calls for baking soda, Epsom salt, citric acid, and corn starch in addition to the oils.

Butters: If you want to make luxurious body butters, you'll need to use natural butters like shea butter, mango butter, or cocoa butter. That said, it's a bit of a specialty ingredient and you might not need it keep it on hand otherwise.

Tools

Several of the spells in part four of this book call for the use of special tools. You don't have to go out and buy all of these right away, but all of the following tools will be helpful to have on your oil magic journey. You may want to dedicate some of these specifically for magical use, although that's completely optional.

Cotton: Cotton balls, cotton cloth, and cotton pouches are all good to have on hand. Cotton balls made of 100 percent cotton make great passive diffusers, and you can wrap them in squares of cotton cloth to make charm bags. Since cotton is a natural fiber, it won't degrade in the presence of oils. You can also use silk, rayon, wool, bamboo, or other 100 percent natural fibers.

Spell candles: Beeswax chime candles are my personal favorite, but other waxes and different shapes will work, too. Be sure they are not scented so they won't be competing with the aromas of your essential oils.

Small knife: This is technically optional, but if you have a small knife dedicated to magical use, you'll find many uses for it, from candle carving to foraging and beyond.

Crystals: These are also optional for oil magic, but crystals and oils pair well. You can use crystals indirectly with oils to charge them, or you can add gem chips to your potions. If you use gem chips, be sure to only use nontoxic crystals with a Mohs' scale hardness of 6 or more. See the spells in part four for specific suggestions.

Oil jewelry: Any jewelry can be anointed with oils, but aromatherapy jewelry such as oil keeper pendants and diffuser necklaces are uniquely suited for oil charms.

Journals: Some spells specifically call for enchanted journals with oil magic, but you may also want to keep a journal with notes on all the blends, recipes, and spells you try.

Mirror: Mirrors are helpful tools for capturing moonlight and aiding affirmation work.

Double boiler: While there are other options for melting and mixing balms, body butters, and salves, a double boiler is ideal.

Molds: You can make bath bombs without molds, but if you want them to be pretty, uniform shapes or you want to make them often, add these to your toolkit.

Electric mixer: You'll really only need this if you want to make body butters, and even then, you *could* use a whisk (and a lot of elbow grease), but it's very nice to have—besides, it's helpful for cooking and baking, too.

PART III

IN THIS PART, we'll explore more closely the properties—both magical and mundane—of the 30 most-used essential oils in this book. From A to Z (or, well, Basil to Ylang Ylang), we'll cover basic correspondences, herbal lore, the magical intentions for which each oil is best suited, mundane applications for each oil, tips for blending, and any precautions you need to be aware of when working with your oils. By the end of this section, you'll know which oils are best for blessing and banishing, for protection and purification, for love and lust, for happiness and healing, for wealth and wellness, and for boosting your magic and manifestation! Furthermore, you'll know whether Lemon or Orange is better for outdoor use, what to do when your bottle of Ginger runs dry, and which oil is known as the Swiss Army knife of essential oils. You can use this section to learn more about why each oil was selected for each spell in part four or use it as a guide to formulating your own potions and magical preparations.

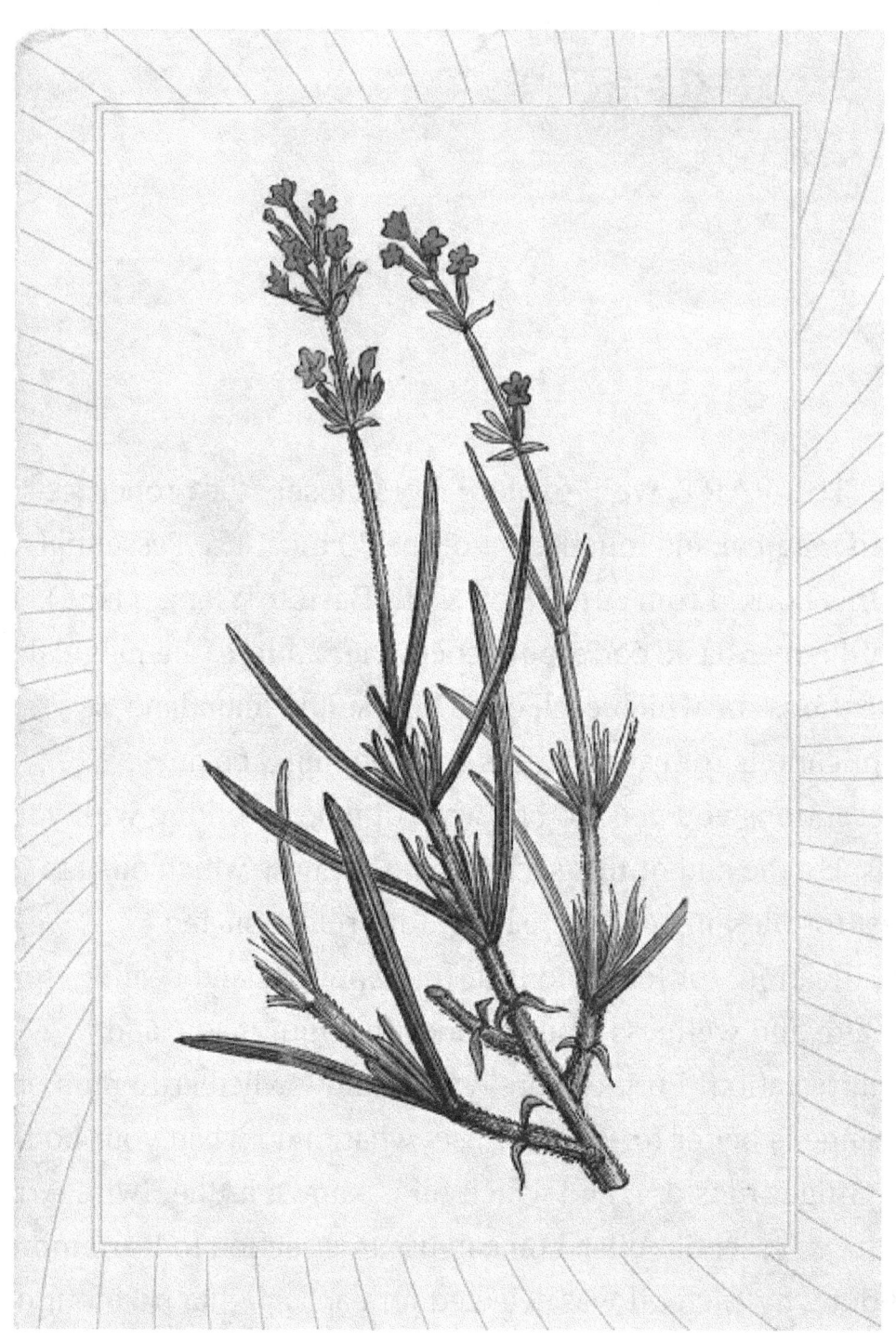

CHAPTER 6
30 Magic Essential Oils

Basil

COMMON NAME: Basil, sweet basil

LATIN NAME: *Ocimum basilicum*

FOLK NAME: Royal Herb, St. Joseph's Wort, Devil Plant

POLARITY: Masculine

MAGICAL INTENTIONS: Love, money, focus, clarity, happiness, attraction, manifestation

PLANETARY RULER: Mars

ELEMENTAL RULER: Fire

DESCRIPTION: If you've ever had bruschetta, caprese, or pesto, you probably know and love the familiar smell of basil. The name "basil" comes from the Latin *basilius* and Greek *basilikon*, both referring to kings, perhaps because it was used in royal perfumery. Basil is also said to have been discovered along with the cross of the crucifixion. But basil is not just associated with Jesus; it has also been called "Devil Plant" by the Greeks and Romans who believed that it was necessary to curse and yell at the earth while planting basil seeds if they were to grow. And if you're wondering whether the phonetic connection to "basilisk" is a coincidence, it's not. Basil was thought to be the antidote to the venom of the mythical basilisk. As if this weren't enough, basil has also come to be associated with love and money, and the ability to attract both.

MAGICAL USES: Though its lore is complex, three magical uses for basil stand out strong. The first is for enhancing clarity of mind and inner vision. Make an inhaler with Basil, Black Spruce, and Clary Sage to see clearly in your mind's eye and make more confident decisions based on your intuition. The second and third magical uses are as an attractant for love and for money. Spray your place of business with a Basil spell spray to attract customers, or wear an aromatherapy locket with Basil and Geranium to attract a lover. Basil essential oil is a key ingredient in both love spells (Like a Moth to a Flame) and prosperity spells (Make It Rain).

OTHER USES: Basil essential oil is prized for its uplifting, energizing, and clarifying aroma. It is sometimes used for support with occasional head tension and may provide support during a menstrual cycle.

PRECAUTIONS: Possible skin sensitizer; dilute appropriately. May not be appropriate for use during pregnancy.

BLENDS WELL WITH: Bergamot, Black Pepper, Black Spruce, Cedarwood, Chamomile, Citronella, Clary Sage, Frankincense, Geranium, Ginger, Grapefruit, Jasmine, Lavender, Lemon, Lemongrass, Neroli, Orange, Palmarosa, Peppermint, Rose

SUBSTITUTE WITH: Black Pepper, Frankincense, Grapefruit, Lemon, Orange, Rose, Rosemary, Spearmint, Tangerine

Black Pepper

COMMON NAME: Pepper

LATIN NAME: *Piper nigrum*

POLARITY: Masculine

MAGICAL INTENTIONS: Banishing, courage, passion, protection, prosperity, strength, vital energy

PLANETARY RULER: Mars

ELEMENTAL RULER: Fire

DESCRIPTION: Black pepper's powerful scent has made it a favorite in the kitchen for at least four thousand years. In fact, it was so highly valued as a spice that it was also used as a valuable currency in ancient Greece and Rome. If you had to describe black pepper's vibe in one word, it might be "stimulating." Physically, it stimulates sensation and is thought by many to stimulate enhanced circulation and metabolism. Energetically, it stimulates physical and mental energy, creative energy, income and economic activity. It is this stimulating energy that creates an energetic defense as well.

MAGICAL USES: Use Black Pepper oil in protective magic designed to keep unwanted spirits and energies at bay (Front Door Defense; Auric Protection Pendant). You can make a roller or a spray with Black Pepper oil and apply it to thresholds, locks, and the soles of your shoes, or use it to anoint and charge protective charms such as the evil eye, the hamsa, and stones like black tourmaline. Salt and pepper, the most fundamental seasoning blend there is, harmonizes absorbent and deflective protection for a powerful charm (Four Corners Fortification). Black Pepper can also be used to magically stimulate mental and physical energy. Make a charm bag from a Black Pepper–infused cotton ball wrapped in a square of red cotton and carry it in your pocket when you need some pep (-per!) in your step, or hang it from the rearview mirror of your car during long drives. When you require a boost of courage, inhale the strengthening aroma of Black Pepper before undertaking the task at hand.

OTHER USES: Black Pepper oil is prized for its antioxidant properties and is sometimes used to support circulation and a healthy immune system.

PRECAUTIONS: Black Pepper is a powerful warming oil and potential sensitizer; dilute appropriately.

BLENDS WELL WITH: Bergamot, Black Spruce, Cardamom, Cedarwood, Clary Sage, Clove, Frankincense, Geranium, Juniper, Lavender, Lime, Myrrh, Orange, Oregano, Nutmeg, Rose, Rosemary, Sage, Tea Tree, Thyme, Vetiver

SUBSTITUTE WITH: Cinnamon, Clove, Ginger, Myrrh, Oregano, Peppermint, Tea Tree

Black Spruce

COMMON NAME: Black spruce, bog spruce, swamp spruce

LATIN NAME: *Picea mariana*

POLARITY: Androgynous

MAGICAL INTENTIONS: Grounding, focus, clarity, healing, expansion, cleansing, protection

PLANETARY RULERS: Moon, Earth

ELEMENTAL RULER: Air

DESCRIPTION: Black spruce is native to North America and is found all over Canada, but other varieties of spruce are similar and found throughout Europe and America. Spruce is traditionally associated with protection, peace, and healing. In ancient Greece, spruce was dedicated to the goddess Artemis, maiden goddess of the Moon and the hunt. Among the Hopi people of the southwestern United States, it is believed that a wise and powerful medicine man turned himself into a spruce tree. To the Salish people of the Pacific Northwest, the spruce is considered to be a symbol of good luck. It is also often used as a Christmas tree. The essential oil is steam distilled from the evergreen leaves. Its invigorating aroma is energetically expansive and stimulating while also being relaxing and grounding.

MAGICAL USES: Include Black Spruce in your workings for cleansing, protection, and blessing (Sacred Space Spray), and diffuse it in your home to bring the expansive enchantment of the forest indoors (Clear the Air). Add it to charms for good luck and good vibes and call upon its magic to clarify your intuition and help you know how to act upon your inner knowings (Aura of Extrasensory Perception; Get Intuit Anywhere).

OTHER USES: Black Spruce is sometimes used by folk practitioners for respiratory and circulatory support and to enhance the appearance of healthy skin.

PRECAUTIONS: None known.

BLENDS WELL WITH: Bergamot, Black Pepper, Chamomile, Citronella, Eucalyptus, Frankincense, Lavender, Jasmine, Lemon, Lime, Neroli, Orange, Petitgrain, Rose, Rosemary, Spearmint, Tangerine, Thyme, Vetiver, Wintergreen, Ylang Ylang

SUBSTITUTE WITH: Blue Spruce, Cypress, Fir, Frankincense, Juniper, Pine, Rosemary, White Spruce

Cardamom

COMMON NAME: Queen of Spices

LATIN NAME: *Elettaria cardamomum*

POLARITY: Feminine

MAGICAL INTENTIONS: Warmth, love, attraction, passion, abundance, joy, creativity

PLANETARY RULER: Venus

ELEMENTAL RULER: Water

DESCRIPTION: Known as the Queen of Spices, Cardamom is one of the most luxurious and delightful aromas there is. The essential oil is distilled from the seeds of the plant, which traditionally are included in chai tea, garam masala, and brewed with coffee in the Middle East to enhance both the flavor and the energetic benefits bestowed by the beverage. It is the third most costly of the spices (after saffron and vanilla), but because the seeds are so rich in essential oil, the oil is not especially expensive.

MAGICAL USES: Cardamom has long been credited with the ability to stimulate lust, passion, and desire, and you will find it included as an ingredient in several love spells in this book (Like a Moth to a Flame; Lovers' Massage Oil), for starters. Its expense and its luxurious aroma have led to an association with wealth and abundance as well, so you'll find it called for in spells like Pocket Pyrite and Abundance Mindset Inhaler. Patchouli, Tangerine, and Cardamom is one of my favorite diffuser blends for infusing a space with love, joy, optimism, a sense of abundance, and all-around good vibes.

OTHER USES: The ancient Egyptians chewed Cardamom seeds to clean their teeth, and the oil is popular in folk remedies today to support tooth and gum health. Cardamom oil is also sometimes used to support a healthy digestive system. Try it in the Happy Tummy Roller after a heavy meal.

PRECAUTIONS: Dilute appropriately and patch test before use.

BLENDS WELL WITH: Bergamot, Black Pepper, Cedarwood, Clove, Ginger, Jasmine, Neroli, Orange, Palmarosa, Patchouli, Petitgrain, Sandalwood, Tangerine, Vetiver, Ylang Ylang

SUBSTITUTE WITH: Cassia, Ginger

Cassia

COMMON NAME: Cassia, false cinnamon, Chinese cinnamon

LATIN NAME: *Cinnamomum cassia*

POLARITY: Masculine

MAGICAL INTENTIONS: Prosperity, protection, warmth, healing, comfort, courage, arousal

PLANETARY RULERS: Jupiter, Mercury, Sun

ELEMENTAL RULER: Fire

DESCRIPTION: While closely related to true cinnamon, cassia is its own plant native to central China. You may be more familiar with it than you think, since much of what is sold in North American grocery stores as "cinnamon" is in fact cassia! Both Cassia and Cinnamon oils are distilled from the fragrant bark of the tree. Its scent is warm, spicy, cozy, festive, and uplifting. In Chinese mythology, cassia is associated with immortality.

MAGICAL USES: Cassia's spicy aroma is warm and uplifting, and can help create an aura of comfort, security, joy, and love. Call upon its energy with Patchouli, Cardamom, and Ginger to spice things up in your love life. As a spice oil, it is also ideal for wealth and prosperity magic, and could stand in for Ginger or Clove in just about any spell in chapter 10. As a hot oil, it can be used in spells for magical protection as well. You'll find it as an ingredient in Sacred Space Spray, Death's Own Cloak, and Going Away Party. Finally, Cassia can also be used to give any spell a bit of a kick and throw some extra fuel on the fire of your intentions.

OTHER USES: In folk practice, Cassia oil is sometimes used to support healthy digestive and immune systems.

PRECAUTIONS: Cassia is considered a hot oil and may irritate sensitive skin; dilute appropriately. May not be appropriate for use during pregnancy.

BLENDS WELL WITH: Bergamot, Black Pepper, Cardamom, Clove, Frankincense, Ginger, Lemon, Neroli, Nutmeg, Orange, Ylang Ylang

SUBSTITUTE WITH: Cinnamon, Clove, Nutmeg

Cedarwood

COMMON NAME: Atlas cedar

LATIN NAME: *Cedrus atlantica*

POLARITY: Masculine

MAGICAL INTENTIONS: Peace, rest, healing, strength, discipline, spirituality, protection

PLANETARY RULERS: Sun, Mercury

ELEMENTAL RULERS: Fire, air

DESCRIPTION: Hailing from Lebanon, the wood of the cedar tree is rich in fragrant oil, the aroma of which has long been thought to repel pests as well as being prized for spiritual use. For this reason, cedar chests have historically been used for storing and protecting precious goods. Many tree oils, such as Juniper and Black Spruce, are typically distilled from the leaves, but high-quality Cedarwood oil is distilled from the fragrant wood of the cedar tree. Its scent is warm, woodsy, and gentle.

MAGICAL USES: In addition to its protective powers, the aroma of Cedarwood promotes spirituality, balance, and all-around good vibes. Use it for rites of blessing and purification, and to support spiritual discipline. Cedarwood may also be helpful in magical workings to banish nightmares, unblock energy centers (chakras), heighten clairvoyance, and bring harmony and balance to any space, to your life in general, or to the manifestation of any intention. Cedarwood can be used in place of Sandalwood in No More Nightmares Pillow Spray, and you can add a few drops of Cedarwood oil to a tarot or oracle deck box for extra spiritual protection. Include Cedarwood in a custom blend to help you stay on track toward achieving your goals.

OTHER USES: Cedarwood is often used to support peaceful sleep and relaxation. It is also sometimes applied for skin support, to enhance the appearance of thick, healthy hair, and is a common ingredient in natural insect repellents.

PRECAUTIONS: Cedarwood oil may irritate sensitive skin; dilute accordingly. May not be appropriate for use during pregnancy.

BLENDS WELL WITH: Bergamot, Cassia, Chamomile, Cinnamon, Clary Sage, Frankincense, Helichrysum, Lavender, Lemon, Palmarosa, Patchouli, Petitgrain, Rose, Rosemary, Sandalwood, Vetiver

SUBSTITUTE WITH: Sandalwood, Vetiver, Patchouli, Frankincense

Chamomile

COMMON NAME: German chamomile, Roman chamomile

LATIN NAME: *Matricaria recutita, Chamaemelum nobile*

FOLK NAME: Blood of Hestia, Ground Apple, Maythe

POLARITY: Androgynous

MAGICAL INTENTIONS: Calming, healing, wealth, cheer, uplifting, cleansing, exorcism, release, love, blessing, luck, money

PLANETARY RULERS: Sun, Moon

ELEMENTAL RULERS: Fire, water

DESCRIPTION: Two plants known as chamomile are popular as essential oils—Roman chamomile (*Chamaemelum nobile*) and German chamomile, sometimes called blue chamomile (*Matricaria recutita*). German Chamomile oil has a distinctive blue color from the constituent chamazulene, which is created during the distillation process, and the two oils have slightly different therapeutic properties, but their magical properties are similar enough to be considered as one. Chamomile is both solar and lunar, fiery and watery, masculine and feminine in its magical nature. Its bright and cheery appearance brings to the mind the Sun and all that goes along with it—gold, money, abundance, luck, success, hope, good vibes, and good fortune. Gamblers and fortune hunters have historically washed their hands with chamomile to attract money and bring good luck in financial dealings. Simultaneously, its relaxing aroma and soothing properties have long caused it to be associated with the gentle loving and healing energy of the Moon. This combination of lunar healing and solar uplifting energy makes chamomile ideal for cleansing, banishing, and exorcism magic. The piercing solar energy drives out darkness and negativity while the gentle lunar energy soothes and heals the damage done.

MAGICAL USES: Chamomile wards dark and negative energy while enhancing relaxation, making it a key ingredient in No More Nightmares Pillow Spray. Include it in spells to inspire healing rest and beauty sleep (Rest and Recover Roller; Summon the Sandman), or to encourage an inner state of peace and optimism (Inner Peace Inhaler). To exorcise and banish negative energy while physically cleansing your home, add a few drops of Chamomile to a natural household cleaner or a homemade vinegar rinse. Good Fortune Fizz calls for Chamomile for its associations with luck, money, and healing. Add a few drops each of Chamomile, Basil, and Lemon essential oils to unscented hand soap to make a money-drawing hand wash, attract abundance, and improve your fortune.

OTHER USES: Chamomile is commonly used for skin support and to encourage sleep and relaxation.

PRECAUTIONS: Avoid this oil if you are taking blood thinners.

BLENDS WELL WITH: Basil, Bergamot, Black Spruce, Blue Tansy, Cedarwood, Citronella, Clary Sage, Grapefruit, Jasmine, Lavender, Lemon, Lemongrass, Myrrh, Neroli, Palmarosa, Palo Santo, Patchouli, Rose, Sage, Tangerine, Thyme, Vetiver, Ylang Ylang

SUBSTITUTE WITH: Cedarwood, Clary Sage, Davana, Eucalyptus, Geranium, Ginger, Helichrysum, Lavender

Citronella

LATIN NAME: *Cymbopogon nardus*

POLARITY: Masculine

MAGICAL INTENTIONS: Cleansing, clearing, purification, protection, motivation, uplifting, psychic awareness

PLANETARY RULERS: Sun, Mercury

ELEMENTAL RULER: Air

DESCRIPTION: Citronella is a type of lemongrass. The various species of *Cymbopogon* are native to tropical regions of Asia, Africa, and Australia. Magically, citronella (*Cymbopogon nardus*) and lemongrass (*Cymbopogon citratus*) are virtually interchangeable, but practically, lemongrass is popular primarily for culinary use whereas citronella is considered too unpalatable to be edible. For cleansing, purification, uplifting, and clarity, either works just as well, but personally I find that citronella has stronger protective properties. (Palmarosa is another gentler type of lemongrass that smells somewhat of rose and can be substituted in many magical applications for either citronella, lemongrass, or rose.)

MAGICAL USES: Citronella is a powerful energy cleanser and can be used to magically purify and uplift the energy of a space by infusing it with piercing solar energy (sunlight both uplifts and drives out dark energy). Diffuse a blend of Citronella, Geranium, and Peppermint to cleanse a space of stagnant and negative energy and fill it with good vibes. Clear the Air is a variation on this idea and calls for Citronella as the primary ingredient. Its purifying properties lend Citronella (and other species of *Cymbopogon*) well to intuitive and divinatory work, too, as it can help clear away that which clouds the inner eye. Add a few drops to a Third Eye Anointing Oil or substitute it for an oil you may not have for that recipe. A simpler alternative anointing oil for this purpose could be made from a blend of Citronella and Cedarwood. Speaking of Citronella and Cedarwood, add one or two drops of each to a few cotton balls to keep in your closet or your dresser drawers to grant your clothing extra protection. Make a spray of Citronella and Lavender to freshen up musty fabric, furniture, and more.

OTHER USES: Citronella is best known for its use as a popular ingredient in natural mosquito repelling products such as natural bug spray and citronella candles. It is also used as an air freshener, in skincare, and in natural household cleaners. Various *Cymbopogon* oils can also be added to facial toners.

PRECAUTIONS: Possible skin sensitization (low risk); dilute appropriately.

BLENDS WELL WITH: Basil, Bergamot, Black Spruce, Cedarwood, Clary Sage, Eucalyptus, Geranium, Ginger, Jasmine, Lavender, Lemon, Lemon Verbena, Lemongrass, Lime, Neroli, Orange, Peppermint, Petitgrain, Pine, Rosemary, Sage, Sandalwood, Spearmint, Tea Tree, Ylang Ylang

SUBSTITUTE WITH: Black Spruce, Chamomile, Eucalyptus, Lemon, Lemon Verbena, Lemongrass, Lime, Palmarosa, Peppermint, Tea Tree

Clary Sage

LATIN NAME: *Salvia sclarea*

FOLK NAME: Clear-Eye

POLARITY: Feminine

MAGICAL INTENTIONS: Clarity, focus, healing, soothing, divination, visions, intuition, balance, euphoria

PLANETARY RULERS: Moon, Mercury, Venus

ELEMENTAL RULERS: Earth, air, water

DESCRIPTION: Clary sage's modern name is a corruption of its old folk name, Clear-Eye. The essential oil is steam distilled from the leaves and flowering tops of the plant. Its fragrance is heady, herbal, and slightly floral. Clary sage is a close relative of common garden sage (see Sage), but their aromas and uses, both magical and mundane, are distinctly different. Its usage in traditional herbalism has led clary sage to be closely associated with women's health, and it is sometimes even called the women's herb.

MAGICAL USES: Magically, clary sage can be used when seeking clarity in the form of mental focus or clear inner vision in divination. Its clarifying nature can also be employed in cleansing and purification spells, although it is more effective at dispelling stagnant energy than distinctly dark or negative energy. Clary sage is a lunar herb and is associated with blood magic, menstruation, pregnancy, childbirth, and more. Women are encouraged to work with clary sage throughout their moon cycle (perhaps keep a moon journal scented with Clary Sage, and whip up a Moontime Roller), although this oil is best avoided during pregnancy. If you use scrying tools such as a bowl, mirror, or crystal ball, make a spell spray with vinegar and Clary Sage oil to cleanse them before and after each use. Store divinatory tools such as pendulums, oracles, and others with a cotton ball scented with drops of Clary Sage, Lavender, and Frankincense. Clary Sage would make a good addition to Prophetic Dreams Pillow Spray or could be substituted for an oil you may not have for that recipe. With its supportive feminine qi, Clary Sage is also associated generally with healing, making it well suited to recipes like Soothing Salve.

OTHER USES: Clary Sage is traditionally popular among women for hormonal support throughout the month. It is believed by many to help balance mood and uplift spirits. It is also often found in hair treatments, and—as its name betrays—was historically used to treat eye problems.

PRECAUTIONS: Not recommended for use during pregnancy. While inhalation of Clary Sage oil is known for its euphoric effects, inhalation in excess may cause headaches and is best avoided; temperance is key.

BLENDS WELL WITH: Bergamot, Black Pepper, Black Spruce, Blue Tansy, Cedarwood, Chamomile, Coriander, Cypress, Frankincense, Geranium, Grapefruit, Jasmine, Juniper, Lavender, Lemon, Lime, Neroli, Patchouli, Petitgrain, Rose, Sandalwood, Tangerine, Ylang Ylang

SUBSTITUTE WITH: Chamomile, Frankincense, Jasmine, Lavender

Clove

COMMON NAME: Clove, clove bud

LATIN NAME: *Syzygium aromaticum*

POLARITY: Masculine

MAGICAL INTENTIONS: Protection, banishing, prosperity, warmth, love, courage

PLANETARY RULER: Jupiter

ELEMENTAL RULER: Fire

DESCRIPTION: Clove oil is steam distilled from the dried flower buds of the clove tree, which is native to the northern Moluccan Islands of Indonesia. Its aroma is warm, spicy, and invigorating. You may recognize it as a key ingredient in pumpkin pie spice. Clove has an ORAC (oxygen radical absorbance capacity) value of over 300,000, making it one of the highest—if not the highest—antioxidant foods known to humans.

MAGICAL USES: Magically, Clove has strong protective properties and can be used to set and reinforce magical boundaries, such as in Four Corners Fortification or Auric Protection Pendant. Its aroma is appropriate for use in love spells, especially in combination with orange; the pair would make a fine candle dressing oil for a variation on Like a Moth to a Flame. Like other warming spice oils, Clove is also associated with wealth and abundance. As such, you'll find it called for in prosperity charms such as Gratitude Journal and Pocket Pyrite.

OTHER USES: Clove oil is frequently found in dental care products to help ease discomfort due to its eugenol content, and this same constituent is useful in the case of ant infestations. It is extremely high in antioxidants and is also sometimes used for immune support.

PRECAUTIONS: Possible skin sensitivity; dilute appropriately. Consult with your doctor before use during pregnancy.

BLENDS WELL WITH: Basil, Bergamot, Black Pepper, Black Spruce, Cassia, Cedarwood, Cinnamon, Frankincense, Geranium, Ginger, Helichrysum, Jasmine, Lavender, Lemon, Myrrh, Nutmeg, Orange, Patchouli, Rose, Rosemary, Tangerine, Ylang Ylang

SUBSTITUTE WITH: Cassia, Cinnamon, Ginger, Nutmeg

Eucalyptus

COMMON NAME: Blue gum tree, narrow-leaved peppermint, eurabbie

LATIN NAME: *Eucalyptus globulus, E. radiata, E. bicostata*

POLARITY: Androgynous

MAGICAL INTENTIONS: Cleansing, clearing, expansive, flow, harmony, healing

PLANETARY RULERS: Moon, Mercury

ELEMENTAL RULERS: Water, air

DESCRIPTION: There are hundreds of species of eucalyptus, several of which are used in aromatherapy and can be incorporated in the practice of oil magic. Their aromas and qi may differ slightly—some may smell more citrusy and uplifting, some more minty and refreshing—but they have more similarities than differences. If you happen to possess several Eucalyptus oils, you may choose one over another for a particular application. For example, I find Eucalyptus Blue gentler and more feminine, and prefer it in many diffuser blends, whereas Eucalyptus Globulus is more masculine, has more kick to it, and is the oil I reach for when I really want to clear things up quickly. However, picking just one to work with across all applications will serve just as well—they are largely interchangeable. Eucalyptus is an evergreen tree that is native to Australia but now found all over the world. The essential oil is steam distilled from the silvery leaves.

MAGICAL USES: One needs only to inhale the aroma of Eucalyptus to experience its cleansing properties. It is immediately palpable in the somatic senses as well as the spirit and mind. To take full advantage of this, let a few drops of Eucalyptus oil fall onto the corner of your shower floor. The steam in your shower will be infused with its invigorating aroma and provide, along with the flowing water, a full cleansing of your spirit and mind. It would likewise be a great addition to the diffuser spell Clear the Air, and you'll notice its protective properties called upon in Death's Own Cloak. These same powers make it helpful in healing spells like Just Breathe and would lend it well to a purification spray (think Citronella, Eucalyptus, Rosemary, and Lavender) you could use all throughout your home, in your car, on your sacred tools, and on yourself and anyone else who needs a good energy cleanse. You could even add drops of Eucalyptus to your natural household cleaners to give them a boost.

OTHER USES: Eucalyptus is familiar as an ingredient in many cough drops and vapor rubs. It is often used for respiratory support in all manner of ways.

PRECAUTIONS: Possible skin sensitivity; dilute appropriately.

BLENDS WELL WITH: Bay Laurel, Bergamot, Cedarwood, Chamomile, Clove, Coriander, Cypress, Geranium, Ginger, Grapefruit, Juniper, Lavender, Lemon, Lime, Marjoram, Orange, Peppermint, Pine, Rose, Rosemary, Tangerine, Thyme

SUBSTITUTE WITH: Peppermint, Tea Tree, Wintergreen

Frankincense

COMMON NAME: Frankincense, Sacred Frankincense

LATIN NAME: *Boswellia carterii, B. sacra*

FOLK NAME: Olibanum, Incense Tree

POLARITY: Masculine

MAGICAL INTENTIONS: Purification, divination, grounding, healing, wealth, prosperity

PLANETARY RULER: Sun

ELEMENTAL RULERS: Air, fire

DESCRIPTION: Frankincense, the resin of trees from the genus *Boswellia* and the essential oil distilled from it, has been in use for spiritual, magical, and medicinal purposes for thousands of years. Historically, frankincense was gifted to kings at their birth, including at the birth of Jesus, because it was believed to have the ability to cure any ailment and thus was considered more valuable than even gold. Frankincense resin is obtained by tapping trees repeatedly in the same spot. The resin is then steam distilled into essential oil form. There are aromatic and functional differences between different species of frankincense, but you can always start with the one you feel drawn to and add to your collection later. Throughout this book, Sacred Frankincense (*B. sacra*) may replace Frankincense (*B. carterii*) if you prefer. I find Sacred Frankincense to be generally more powerful for magical use, but it is also more costly.

MAGICAL USES: Frankincense has long been used to cleanse and purify sacred space. Diffuse it wherever you need to clear out dark or stagnant energy.

Going Away Party is a riff on this idea, but more mobile than a diffuser. You can also use it to purify your own energy, such as with Protection Polish. Clearing space within yourself and your life is necessary for manifesting your desires, making Frankincense helpful in manifestation magic such as the love-drawing spell Like a Moth to a Flame. That, plus its considerable value, lends it to spells of wealth and prosperity, such as Liquid Gold Body Wash and Midas Touch Body Butter. Frankincense is also thought to stimulate the pineal gland and open the third eye, which makes it ideal for inclusion in divination spells. As such, you'll find it in Third Eye Anointing Oil, Soothsayer's Soak, Rose Runes, and several other spells in chapter 11. Finally, Frankincense's long-standing associations with health and wellness lend it to a selection of healing spells in chapter 9, including Soothing Salve and Miracle Massage Oil.

OTHER USES: Historically, frankincense was believed to cure any ailment. While this may be a little extreme, its uses are indeed many. It is helpful in skincare to reduce the appearance of fine lines and as an addition to your moisturizer. It is also used to aid meditation and focus, and is being studied for possible applications to cancer.

PRECAUTIONS: None known.

BLENDS WELL WITH: Angelica, Basil, Bergamot, Black Spruce, Cassia, Cedarwood, Cinnamon, Clary Sage, Davana, Geranium, Ginger, Helichrysum, Jasmine, Juniper, Lavender, Orange, Patchouli, Rose, Rosemary, Sage, Sandalwood, Tangerine, Vetiver, Ylang Ylang

SUBSTITUTE WITH: Black Spruce, Elemi, Helichrysum, Myrrh, Palo Santo, Sandalwood

Geranium

COMMON NAME: Rose geranium

LATIN NAME: *Pelargonium graveolens*

POLARITY: Feminine

MAGICAL INTENTIONS: Love, fertility, friendship, peace, protection, harmony, hex-breaking

PLANETARY RULER: Venus

ELEMENTAL RULER: Water

DESCRIPTION: A little trivia: The plants that bear the genus *Geranium* are commonly known as cranesbills, whereas the plants commonly known as geraniums are in fact of the genus *Pelargonium*. In the world of essential oils, aromatherapy, and oil magic, when you hear the word "geranium," it is safe to assume we are speaking of *Pelargonium graveolens* or another member of that genus. That said, geraniums are bred for their scent, and *Pelargonium graveolens* is known for its green, rosy aroma that cleanses and uplifts. The essential oil is typically steam distilled from the leaves of the plant.

MAGICAL USES: Geranium has energy that is very similar to that of Rose, only I would describe it as softer, milder, gentler, and less extreme. Both are helpful in matters of love, but whereas Rose may be applied to romance and passion, Geranium is more appropriate for friendship, solidifying long-term relationships, and sowing peace. Diffuse Geranium to resolve disagreements among fellows and sow friendship between strangers. Its gentle, loving energy makes it appropriate for the Self-Love Mirror Spell and Yummy Love Scrub. Its positivity is so strong and cleansing that it is considered one of the primary plant allies for hex-breaking and curse prevention. It works as both a shield, like a force field of good vibes, and a solution, neutralizing malicious energy where it stands. As such, you'll find it in Roll-On Energy Shield, Front Door Defense, and other protection spells. It is especially good for protecting the cozy, happy energy of a home.

OTHER USES: Geranium oil is used in skincare, to discourage pests, and for mood support, among other things.

PRECAUTIONS: Possible skin sensitivity; dilute appropriately.

BLENDS WELL WITH: Basil, Bergamot, Black Spruce, Cedarwood, Chamomile, Clary Sage, Clove, Ginger, Grapefruit, Jasmine, Juniper, Lavender, Lemon, Lime, Neroli, Orange, Palmarosa, Peppermint, Rose, Rosemary, Sage, Sandalwood, Tangerine, Thyme, Ylang Ylang

SUBSTITUTE WITH: Chamomile, Cistus, Davana, Eucalyptus, Lavender, Petitgrain, Rose

Ginger

LATIN NAME: *Zingiber officinale*

POLARITY: Masculine

MAGICAL INTENTIONS: Warmth, love, passion, healing, wealth, prosperity, vitality

PLANETARY RULER: Mars

ELEMENTAL RULER: Fire

DESCRIPTION: Ginger was first cultivated somewhere in Asia, although as it happened over four thousand years ago, no one knows just exactly where. Though ginger flowers are spectacular, it is the root (or really, the rhizome) that we use, know, and love. Ginger root has been a favorite for centuries for its applications in cooking and herbal medicine. Confucius himself ate ginger with every meal—enough to add flavor and support digestion, but not so much as to warm the body excessively. The essential oil is steam distilled from the roots.

MAGICAL USES: Ginger's magical uses are many and potent. First and foremost, Ginger can be used to add power and zest to any magical working or practitioner. Add a drop to your moisturizer to jump-start your day and level up your magic. This same principle can be applied in the bedroom, which is why you'll find Ginger called for in love spell preparations such as Lovers' Massage Oil, Love Potion No. 10, and Yummy Love Scrub. Ginger's magical firepower (so to speak) adds a welcome punch to prosperity spells like Minting Money and the Gratitude Journal. As for its applications to health and wellness, you need only read Confucius to know why it's such an important ingredient in the Happy Tummy Roller.

OTHER USES: Ginger is frequently used for digestive support, for general wellness, and to heat things up in the bedroom.

PRECAUTIONS: Possible skin sensitivity; dilute appropriately. Consult a doctor before use if you are taking any blood-thinning medication.

BLENDS WELL WITH: Bergamot, Black Pepper, Cardamom, Cassia, Cedarwood, Cinnamon, Clove, Coriander, Frankincense, Geranium, Grapefruit, Helichrysum, Jasmine, Juniper, Lemon, Lime, Neroli, Orange, Palmarosa, Patchouli, Rose, Sandalwood, Spearmint, Vetiver, Ylang Ylang

SUBSTITUTE WITH: Cardamom, Peppermint, Spearmint

Helichrysum

COMMON NAME: Italian strawflower, curry plant

LATIN NAME: *Helichrysum italicum*

FOLK NAME: Immortelle, Everlasting

POLARITY: Feminine

MAGICAL INTENTIONS: Healing, intuition, preservation, divination, creativity, cleansing, clarity

PLANETARY RULERS: Sun, Jupiter, Mercury

ELEMENTAL RULERS: Fire, water, air

DESCRIPTION: "Helichrysum" is derived from Greek words meaning "golden sun," referring to the appearance of its golden-yellow flowers. The flowers retain their fragrance and appearance even once dried, earning them the nicknames Everlasting and Immortelle. Helichrysum is beloved by many for its distinct spicy-sweet (perhaps curry-like) scent and the numerous healing properties attributed to it. The flower tops are steam distilled to yield the essential oil.

MAGICAL USES: Helichrysum is chiefly useful in healing magic, and you'll find it called for in both Soothing Salve and Miracle Massage Oil, where you may indeed find it to perform miraculously. It can also be used in the healing of psychic wounds by helping to clear away energy and release thought forms that are no longer needed, opening up space and inviting more positive and productive thoughts and things to take their place. It follows that Helichrysum could be an appropriate choice for energy cleansing as a precursor to protective magic, as well as wealth and prosperity magic.

Helichrysum is psychically stimulating, and may be called on to aid with divinatory work, such as in Third Eye Anointing Oil, the scented Olfactory Oracle, and Prophetic Dreams Pillow Spray. Finally, Helichrysum is connected with the mysteries of birth, death, and rebirth, and may be called on in magical matters connected to these.

OTHER USES: Helichrysum is frequently used to support the skin in its natural healing process. It can also be used to support emotional healing.

PRECAUTIONS: None known.

BLENDS WELL WITH: Bergamot, Black Pepper, Chamomile, Clary Sage, Clove, Cypress, Frankincense, Geranium, Ginger, Grapefruit, Juniper, Lavender, Lemon, Neroli, Orange, Patchouli, Rose, Rosemary, Tea Tree, Thyme, Vetiver, Ylang Ylang

SUBSTITUTE WITH: Lavender, Myrrh, Patchouli

Jasmine

COMMON NAME: True jasmine, poet's jasmine

LATIN NAME: *Jasminum officinale*

POLARITY: Feminine

MAGICAL INTENTIONS: Dreams, visions, divination, love, romance, enchantment, calming

PLANETARY RULERS: Moon, Stars

ELEMENTAL RULER: Water

DESCRIPTION: Jasmine flowers are too delicate to survive the process of steam distillation, which destroys key compounds in what would be the essential oil. As such, Jasmine oil is only available as an absolute, which means it is extracted with solvents instead of steam. Carbon dioxide extraction is widely considered to be the best method for extracting Jasmine absolute. Whether or not any solvents remain in the finished product depends on the maker and the technique. Jasmine absolute is extraordinarily fragrant and even one drop can overwhelm a blend (use a toothpick if you need less). However, the enchanting magic of this oil and its aroma are too good to miss. It is my favorite oil for working with the magic of the Moon and stars.

MAGICAL USES: Jasmine's enchanting aroma is ideal for all forms of moon magic and star magic. Anoint yourself with Jasmine when drawing down the moon and at full moon rituals and anoint magical items with Jasmine oil before charging them in the full moonlight. Write down your moon cycle manifestation goals and scent the paper with Jasmine. Diffuse Jasmine on the full moon along with Lemon, Grapefruit, Orange, Neroli, Rose, Sandalwood, Bergamot, Frankincense, Lavender, or Clary Sage. Jasmine has long been associated with love, lust, and romance, and would make a great addition to or substitute in the charm Freyja's Necklace or the diffuser spell In the Mood for Love. Make a glass cleaner for your mirrors with white vinegar and Jasmine to see yourself in a more gentle and loving light. Jasmine's association with divination, nighttime, and relaxation make it a key ingredient in Prophetic Dreams Pillow Spray. You'll also find it in other divination spells such as Inner Eye Illumination and Third Eye Anointing Oil.

OTHER USES: Jasmine has long been believed to have aphrodisiac powers, and is often used for this purpose, as well as to lift the mood and relax the mind and body. It is heavily used in the perfume industry.

PRECAUTIONS: No known precautions, but be very mindful to only purchase pure, authentic Jasmine absolute! The cost to procure this oil has led to the presence of many fakes on the market that are more likely to cause irritation and less likely to possess any sort of magic.

BLENDS WELL WITH: Bergamot, Cassia, Clary Sage, Clove, Coriander, Geranium, Ginger, Grapefruit, Frankincense, Lavender, Lemon, Lemongrass, Melissa, Myrrh, Neroli, Orange, Palmarosa, Patchouli, Petitgrain, Rose, Sandalwood, Spearmint, Ylang Ylang

SUBSTITUTE WITH: Neroli, Sandalwood, Ylang Ylang

Lavender

COMMON NAME: Elf leaf, English lavender

LATIN NAME: *Lavandula angustifolia*

POLARITY: Androgynous

MAGICAL INTENTIONS: Peace, calming, soothing, healing, grounding, love, intuition, dreams

PLANETARY RULERS: Mercury, Moon

ELEMENTAL RULER: Air

DESCRIPTION: Lavender is perhaps the best known, most popular, and most well-loved of all essential oils. Many people, when they think of essential oil, immediately think of Lavender. No list of must-have essential oils is complete without Lavender. If you must start your collection with only one oil, start with Lavender (okay, or maybe Frankincense. It's a close call—don't make me choose). The essential oil is distilled from the fragrant purple flowers and is commonly used in soaps and air fresheners, as well as fougère fragrances. Fougères were originally formulated for women but are now mostly marketed to men; similarly, most magical sources list lavender as a masculine herb, but laymen intuitively classify it as feminine, as do I. For this reason, I have listed it as androgynous. Lavender takes its name from the French word *lavandre*, in turn from the Latin word *lavare*, "to wash," as it has historically been used in soaps of all kinds.

MAGICAL USES: Lavender's roots in washing up are tied to its present use in magic as an energetic cleanser. It is used to purify and consecrate, such as in Sacred Space Spray and Clear the Air. Lavender is also supremely relaxing and is appropriate in spells and potions for relaxing the body (Soothing

Salve; Soothing Soak; Moontime Roller) as well as the mind (Inner Peace Inhaler ; Wash Your Worries Away; Summon the Sandman; Let the Good Times Roll. Its gentle, loving energy lends it well to heart-healing spells such as Self-Love Mirror Spell and Anahata Opening. Finally, its powers of relaxation make it an appropriate choice for quieting the yammering of the conscious mind and inviting the voice of intuition to speak more clearly. As such, you'll find it useful in divination spells like Olfactory Oracle, Inner Eye Illumination, and Prophetic Dreams Pillow Spray, to name a few.

OTHER USES: Lavender is sometimes called the Swiss Army knife of the oil world because it has such a wide range of traditional uses. Lavender was the oil René-Maurice Gattefossé credited with the miraculous healing of his burned arm in 1910. It is beloved by women for support throughout the monthly cycle, and by nearly everyone for purposes of sleep support, skin support, seasonal support . . . the list really does go on and on. It's also extremely popular in household and personal care products from laundry detergent to lash serum.

PRECAUTIONS: No known precautions.

BLENDS WELL WITH: Bergamot, Black Pepper, Black Spruce, Cedarwood, Chamomile, Clary Sage, Clove, Davana, Elemi, Eucalyptus, Frankincense, Geranium, Jasmine, Lemon, Lemongrass, Lime, Myrrh, Neroli, Nutmeg, Orange, Patchouli, Peppermint, Pine, Rose, Rosemary, Sandalwood, Tangerine, Tea Tree, Thyme, Vetiver, Ylang Ylang

SUBSTITUTE WITH: Cedarwood, Chamomile, Clary Sage, Helichrysum, Rosemary, Sandalwood

Lemon

LATIN NAME: *Citrus limon*

POLARITY: Feminine

MAGICAL INTENTIONS: Cleansing, clarity, uplifting, protection, purification, abundance

PLANETARY RULERS: Moon, Sun

ELEMENTAL RULER: Water

DESCRIPTION: Lemon oil is typically cold-pressed from the peels of lemons. This method preserves the true fragrance of lemon but also preserves the furocoumarins that make Lemon and several other citrus oils phototoxic. Steam distillation removes the issue of phototoxicity but also removes much of what makes Lemon oil smell so "lemony."

MAGICAL USES: Lemon is one of the most versatile oils for magical use. It is a wonderful ally for both physical cleaning and spiritual cleansing. You'll find it is a key ingredient in spells like Death's Own Cloak and Front Door Defense, and it makes a fine substitute for Citronella or Lemongrass in cleansing and protection spells. Lemon is also associated with love magic and could be added to or substituted in spells such as Like a Moth to a Flame or Self-Love Mirror Spell. Round and yellow like a gold coin and bearing all the symbolism of abundant fruit, lemons and Lemon oil are also good for wealth and money magic. It could be used in place of (or in addition to) Orange oil in just about any spell in chapter 10. Finally, its associations with clarity lend its powers well to divinatory magic, and it would make a great addition to a spell like Aura of Extrasensory Perception.

OTHER USES: Lemon oil is popularly used in household cleaning products and can be used to remove gummy sticker residue from glass, metal, and ceramic surfaces. Be careful, though—it can also remove paint or wood varnish and dissolve plastic.

PRECAUTIONS: Cold-pressed Lemon oil is phototoxic, which causes increased photosensitivity. Do not apply to skin that will be exposed to sunlight except in very low concentrations of 2 percent or less. Steam-distilled Lemon oil is not phototoxic.

BLENDS WELL WITH: Basil, Bergamot, Black Pepper, Black Spruce, Cedarwood, Citronella, Coriander

SUBSTITUTE WITH: Bergamot, Citronella, Grapefruit, Lemon Verbena, Lemongrass, Lime, Melissa, Tangerine

Myrrh

LATIN NAME: *Commiphora myrrha*

POLARITY: Masculine

MAGICAL INTENTIONS: Protection, spirituality, prosperity, preservation, divination, wealth, purification, banishing

PLANETARY RULERS: Sun, Saturn

ELEMENTAL RULERS: Fire, water

DESCRIPTION: Even those who do not know what myrrh is have surely heard of it, for who cannot recount the three gifts of the Magi to the infant Jesus? They were gold, frankincense, and myrrh—one precious metal and two resin incenses, both of which are now available as two of the most popular and versatile essential oils. Myrrh resin, from which the essential oil is distilled, has a long history as part of the ancient Egyptian embalming process, and as an ingredient in the Jerusalem temple incense. It is also used in Western, Chinese, and Ayurvedic medicine, is mentioned throughout the old and new testaments of the Bible, and is still today used in religious rituals around the world. The sap is bled from the trees and dried into resinous form before being distilled into essential oil form. The name "myrrh" comes from the Arabic word for "bitter" due to the resin's sharp, medicinal taste.

MAGICAL USES: The first of Myrrh's magical properties are purification, banishing, and protection. It is a key ingredient in Roll-On Energy Shield, Protection Polish, Auric Protection Pendant, and many other spells of this type. Anoint locks with Myrrh to add a layer of magical protection and make a spell spray with Myrrh for banishing and energy clearing. Myrrh is also associated with life, longevity, death, and the afterlife, due to its ties to mummification, the crucifixion, and herbal medicine. This makes it appropriate in health and healing spells. Mix up a bubble bath (here) or a moisturizing salve (here) with Frankincense, Myrrh, and other oils of your choice. It is also suitable for divinatory work (Aura of Extrasensory Perception, especially that which involves communicating with the dead (Patchouli and Myrrh are a great combo for this). Its value has also led to an association with wealth and money magic, and Myrrh may aid with manifestation magic as well (Pocket Pyrite; Liquid Gold Body Wash).

OTHER USES: Myrrh is commonly used as a fixative in perfumery. A small amount of Myrrh may be added to a blend to make the more volatile top notes last longer.

PRECAUTIONS: Myrrh is not recommended for pregnant or breastfeeding women.

BLENDS WELL WITH: Black Spruce, Cassia, Cedarwood, Chamomile, Clove, Davana, Frankincense, Geranium, Jasmine, Lavender, Lemon, Orange, Patchouli, Rose, Sandalwood, Tangerine, Vetiver, Ylang Ylang

SUBSTITUTE WITH: Frankincense, Helichrysum, Patchouli, Sandalwood, Vetiver

Nutmeg

LATIN NAME: *Myristica fragrans*

POLARITY: Masculine

MAGICAL INTENTIONS: Love, lust, luck, health, wealth, fidelity, vitality, protection

PLANETARY RULER: Jupiter

ELEMENTAL RULER: Fire

DESCRIPTION: The *Myristica fragrans* tree is an evergreen found mainly in Indonesia and produces not one but two beloved spices—mace, from the seed covering, and nutmeg, from the seed itself. Nutmeg oil is steam distilled from the ground seeds and has a long history of culinary use dating back to prehistoric times.

MAGICAL USES: Like many of the other spice oils, Nutmeg is tied to the element of fire and is associated with matters of love, sex, money, purification, and protection. You'll find it featured in Love Potion No. 10 and the charm Freyja's Necklace to enhance desire and increase attraction. This element of attraction can also be employed in spells to attract money or other desired manifestations. Consider adding Nutmeg to Straw into Gold Hair Oil or the Pocket Pyrite charm. You may also find the energy of Nutmeg helpful when you need to recharge your own magical energy or jump-start your day. It can be substituted for Clove or Cassia or added to any banishing or protection spell, such as Sacred Space Spray or Four Corners Fortification.

OTHER USES: Nutmeg is the primary spice behind the flavor of the yuletide beverage eggnog. Nutmeg essential oil is used in modern times as a food flavoring agent and as an ingredient in toothpastes and cough syrups.

PRECAUTIONS: Use sparingly. May have adverse effects when used in excess. Not recommended during pregnancy.

BLENDS WELL WITH: Bay Laurel, Cardamom, Cassia, Cedarwood, Cinnamon, Clary Sage, Clove, Frankincense, Geranium, Ginger, Lavender, Lime, Orange, Patchouli, Petitgrain, Rose, Rosemary, Tangerine, Vetiver

SUBSTITUTE WITH: Cassia, Cinnamon, Clove, Ginger

Orange

COMMON NAME: Sweet orange

LATIN NAME: *Citrus sinensis*

POLARITY: Androgynous

MAGICAL INTENTIONS: Uplifting, abundance, joy, love, fertility, happiness

PLANETARY RULERS: Sun, Venus

ELEMENTAL RULERS: Fire, water

DESCRIPTION: Orange essential oil is one of the sweetest and most joyful and uplifting oils of all time, and a collection is hardly complete without it. The particular Orange oil in question here is that of the sweet orange, *Citrus sinensis*, which in addition to its other many virtues possesses no phototoxicity and is perfectly safe for topical use with sun exposure. This is also true of Tangerine, which is approximately magically equivalent, although I find Tangerine to be slightly gentler and more feminine in its qi. Bitter Orange (*Citrus aurantium*), on the other hand, is quite phototoxic, although Neroli and Petitgrain, made from the blossoms and wood of *Citrus aurantium*, respectively, are not phototoxic.

MAGICAL USES: Orange uplifts and brings joy, so you'll find it crucial in spells such as Inner Peace Inhaler and Wash Your Worries Away. As a golden fruit, it is a symbol of abundance, and earns its place as the top note in many of the wealth and prosperity spells in this book (Make It Rain; Let the Good Times Roll; Midas Touch Body Butter). Orange is also intensely loving and brings sweetness and inspires love wherever it is used (Self-Love Mirror Spell; Lovers' Massage Oil). Orange and Neroli are both appropriate for love and fertility magic (especially at weddings, and both can be used during pregnancy), and Petitgrain can be called upon to support emotional stability and to magically reinforce and secure the joy that Orange brings.

OTHER USES: Orange oil is most often used in aromatherapy to lift the mood and for emotional support. It is also popular as a flavoring agent and as a joyful top note in perfumery.

PRECAUTIONS: No known precautions.

BLENDS WELL WITH: Citrus oils blend well with just about everything—seriously! You simply *must* try it with Frankincense, Lavender, and Black Spruce, however.

SUBSTITUTE WITH: Tangerine, Neroli, Petitgrain (for topical use anywhere); Bergamot, Grapefruit, Lemon, Lime (not for topical use where the sun shines)

Patchouli

LATIN NAME: *Pogostemon cablin*

FOLK NAME: Pucha-Pat

POLARITY: Feminine

MAGICAL INTENTIONS: Grounding, prosperity, wealth, passion, divination, spirit work, fertility

PLANETARY RULER: Saturn

ELEMENTAL RULER: Earth

DESCRIPTION: This rich and earthy oil is steam distilled from the leaves of the patchouli plant, an herb from the mint family. It is native to the islands of Southeast Asia, and is a traditional component of India ink, as well as a common ingredient in perfumery (especially the class of perfumes known as *chypres*). Both its association with fine fabrics and its earthy smell have led to it being associated with wealth and luxury, and its ties to the element of earth further connect it with matters of birth, death, and rebirth. True Patchouli oil is considered to improve with age.

MAGICAL USES: As one of the earthiest of all essential oils, Patchouli is appropriate for all earth magic. This includes spells for grounding as well as for wealth and prosperity, such as the Abundance Mindset Inhaler, Midas Touch Body Butter, and Good Fortune Fizz. Besides fertility of the wallet, Patchouli is also appropriate for magic surrounding fertility of people. It can be used in manifestation magic of all kinds. The aroma of Patchouli has historically been attributed aphrodisiac properties, which make it well suited for certain types of love magic, such as Goddess Body Wash and Freyja's Necklace. The protective properties that originally lent it to be packaged with textiles for shipping make it appropriate in many forms of protective magic as well, such as the shower scrub spell Protection Polish. Its ties to the earth, birth, death, and rebirth make Patchouli appropriate for spirit work and divination that involves communication with the dead.

OTHER USES: Fresh patchouli leaves were traditionally used to wrap and protect fine silks and other cloth goods from mold and bugs during ocean transport from India.

PRECAUTIONS: Possible skin sensitivity; dilute appropriately. If you are pregnant, nursing, or on medication, consult your physician before use.

BLENDS WELL WITH: Bergamot, Black Pepper, Black Spruce, Cassia, Cedarwood, Cinnamon, Clary Sage, Clove, Frankincense, Geranium, Ginger, Grapefruit, Jasmine, Lavender, Myrrh, Neroli, Orange, Peppermint, Rose, Sandalwood, Tangerine, Vetiver, Ylang Ylang

SUBSTITUTE WITH: Helichrysum, Myrrh, Sandalwood, Vetiver

Peppermint

COMMON NAME: Brandy mint, lamb mint

LATIN NAME: *Mentha piperita*

POLARITY: Masculine

MAGICAL INTENTIONS: Clearing, cleansing, focus, clarity, motivation, energy, boosting, quickening, refreshing, balancing, purification, healing

PLANETARY RULER: Mercury

ELEMENTAL RULER: Air

DESCRIPTION: The same peppermint you know from herbal teas and candy canes is a much-beloved essential oil. It is one of the most popular oils, and one of the first that many novice oil witches acquire—and it's no wonder why! Its uses are many and varied. Its aroma is stimulating and refreshing, and it grows abundantly. In some gardens, peppermint grows *so* abundantly that it is even considered invasive! The essential oil is high in the constituents menthol and eucalyptol, and is steam distilled from the leaves of the herb.

MAGICAL USES: Peppermint's chief magical property is that of clarity and purification. This property lends it well to spells like Just Breathe and would make it a welcome addition to the diffuser spell Clear the Air, the Sacred Space Spray, or the Front Door Defense charm. Peppermint's aroma is mentally stimulating, so you may want to call on its power during meditation or whenever your mind requires refreshment. The abundant nature of peppermint makes its oil a natural addition to wealth and money spells such as Make It Rain and, of course, Minting Money. Lastly, Peppermint is well suited to certain types of healing preparations like Miracle Massage Oil and the Happy Tummy Roller, thanks to its natural constituents.

OTHER USES: Peppermint is frequently used for digestive support, to provide a relieving cooling sensation in areas of occasional discomfort, and to relieve occasional head tension. It is commonly found as an ingredient in natural pest repellents.

PRECAUTIONS: Possible skin sensitivity; dilute appropriately. Do not use Peppermint oil to enable poor eating habits.

BLENDS WELL WITH: Basil, Bergamot, Geranium, Ginger, Grapefruit, Lavender, Lemon, Lime, Orange, Pine, Rosemary, Spearmint, Tangerine, Wintergreen, Ylang Ylang

SUBSTITUTE WITH: Cardamom, Ginger, Spearmint

Rose

COMMON NAME: Rose, damask rose

LATIN NAME: *Rosa damascena*

FOLK NAME: Queen of Flowers

POLARITY: Feminine

MAGICAL INTENTIONS: Love, passion, protection, prosperity, emotional healing, heart-opening

PLANETARY RULER: Venus

ELEMENTAL RULERS: Water, earth

DESCRIPTION: There is a reason the rose is called the Queen of Flowers. Is there any other flower so steeped in enchantment, lore, and tradition as she? From *Romeo and Juliet* to *Beauty and the Beast,* from the virtuous Virgin Mary to the passionate goddess Aphrodite, literature, myth, and magic are brimming with roses. The aroma is incomparable, and the magic potent. The damask rose is a hybrid with centuries-old origins in Asia, and is the type of rose still cultivated today for its fragrance, which is prized for its medicinal, cosmetic, and aromatherapeutic value. The essential oil is steam distilled from the blossoms. Sixty roses are needed to yield a single drop of Rose essential oil, or about 10,000 roses to fill a 5-milliliter bottle—no wonder it is so precious! The price tag may seem extravagant, but once you have worked with true Rose oil, you will never want to go without it. Note that rose is often solvent distilled as an absolute, which does not match the quality of true Rose essential oil and may not be appropriate for therapeutic use. The true essential oil is sometimes called Rose otto.

MAGICAL USES: Rose is a great heart healer, and its long-standing ties to love, matters of the heart, and goddesses like Venus, Aphrodite, and Freyja make it the number one choice for all acts of love magic. You can work without it or substitute it, but you need only use it once to see why it is worth the investment. Rose makes magic in love spells like Goddess Body Wash, Love Potion No. 10, and Aphrodite's Bath. Just as a rose protects its own valuable blossoms with thorns, its energy can lend its protection to you and your valuables (Protection Polish; Auric Protection Pendant). If healing is what you need, its gentle yet potent loving energy would be a welcome addition to a Soothing Salve or Moontime Roller. You may notice a pattern that costly botanicals and expensive oils, by the principles of sympathetic magic, are thought to attract wealth and prosperity. Abundance is apparent in the luxurious petals of the damask rose, and feelings of luxury are inevitable when you slather yourself in Midas Touch Body Butter or care for your luscious locks with Straw into Gold Hair Oil. Finally, rose connects the spiritual to the material, which is why it is perfect for consecrating divinatory tools (Rose Runes).

OTHER USES: Rose oil is extraordinarily popular in skincare and beauty products, as it offers a multitude of benefits to the skin. It is also used to support women's health.

PRECAUTIONS: None known. Dilute appropriately.

BLENDS WELL WITH: Rose oil honestly blends well with just about every other oil. It holds its own and complements a variety of fragrances well. It is very strong, though, and you will often only need one drop of Rose to several of each of the other oils you are using.

SUBSTITUTE WITH: Geranium, Neroli, Palmarosa

Rosemary

LATIN NAME: *Rosmarinus officinalis*

FOLK NAME: Dew of the Sea

POLARITY: Masculine

MAGICAL INTENTIONS: Focus, clarity, memory, cleansing, clearing, awakening, purification

PLANETARY RULER: Sun

ELEMENTAL RULER: Fire

DESCRIPTION: The connection between rosemary and memory is timeless and was even confirmed by a 2017 study published in the *Egyptian Journal of Basic and Applied Sciences*. Rosemary oil is distilled from leaves of the Mediterranean evergreen herb.

MAGICAL USES: Rosemary's magical properties of purification and protection make it an important ingredient in spells like Clear the Air and Death's Own Cloak. Its associations with mental clarity make it an ideal ingredient in spells for divinatory work (Olfactory Oracle; Get Intuit Anywhere). To magically enhance memory, inhale Rosemary both when you are studying or reading up on something and later when you need to recall it. Scent any books, journals, or magazines that you may reference with a drop of Rosemary. Rosemary is also associated with health and beauty. Make a spell spray with Cedarwood, Lavender, and Rosemary, fondly known as Mermaid Spray, and spray it on your scalp daily to tame wild tresses and support the appearance of thick and healthy hair. (Do not use alcohol on hair; use polysorbate 20 instead.) This Mermaid Spray can double as a purification and energy cleansing spray. It is multipurpose enough to merit a spot in your everyday carry-along.

OTHER USES: Rosemary oil is popular as a flavoring agent and for immune support. It is also often found in haircare products to support the appearance of thick and healthy hair.

PRECAUTIONS: Possible skin sensitivity; dilute appropriately. May not be appropriate for use during pregnancy.

BLENDS WELL WITH: Basil, Bergamot, Black Pepper, Cassia, Cedarwood, Cinnamon, Citronella, Clary Sage, Elemi, Eucalyptus, Frankincense, Geranium, Grapefruit, Jasmine, Lavender, Lemon, Lime, Neroli, Orange, Oregano, Peppermint, Petitgrain, Pine, Sage, Tangerine, Tea Tree, Thyme

SUBSTITUTE WITH: Clary Sage, Eucalyptus, Lavender, Sage

Sage

COMMON NAME: Common sage, garden sage, true sage, dalmatian sage, toad

LATIN NAME: *Salvia officinalis*

FOLK NAME: Toad

POLARITY: Masculine

MAGICAL INTENTIONS: Blessing, hallowing, healing, longevity, protection, wealth, wisdom

PLANETARY RULER: Jupiter

ELEMENTAL RULER: Air

DESCRIPTION: A close relative of the magically popular clary sage and white sage, plain old sage is anything but plain. Its aroma is heady, simultaneously herbaceous and spicy with notes of camphor. The oil is steam distilled from the leaves of the herb. Well-loved in the kitchen, common garden sage may become a favorite in your oil apothecary as well. In old coded recipes, "toad" refers to sage. A potion calling for the legs of a toad is really calling for leaves of sage.

MAGICAL USES: Sage is probably best known among witches for its use in hallowing or blessing a space. Many use it for cleansing and clearing as well, but in my opinion, it should be paired with a stronger energetic cleansing herb or oil such as Citronella, Black Spruce, Peppermint, Juniper, Lemon, or Myrrh, and called upon primarily to bless, hallow, and protect energy, such as in Sacred Space Spray or Going Away Party. Sage can also be included in spells to nurture and develop wisdom. Diffuse it with Frankincense during meditation for this purpose.

OTHER USES: Sage has been traditionally associated with longevity. In Britain there is an old saying: *He that would live for aye* [forever] *must eat sage in May.* Sage and its essential oil have traditionally been used to support memory and general physical and mental health.

PRECAUTIONS: Use in moderation. Best avoided during pregnancy. Not appropriate for use by people with seizure disorders. Hot oil; dilute appropriately.

BLENDS WELL WITH: Bay Laurel, Bergamot, Cassia, Cinnamon, Clary Sage, Frankincense, Geranium, Ginger, Grapefruit, Jasmine, Lavender, Lemon, Lime, Neroli, Orange, Palo Santo, Patchouli, Petitgrain, Rosemary, Sandalwood, Tea Tree, Thyme, Vetiver, Ylang Ylang

SUBSTITUTE WITH: Bay Laurel, Clary Sage, Rosemary, Juniper, Lavender, Palo Santo, Myrrh

Sandalwood

COMMON NAME: Indian sandalwood, royal Hawaiian sandalwood, Australian sandalwood

LATIN NAME: *Santalum album, S. paniculatum, S. spicatum*

POLARITY: Androgynous

MAGICAL INTENTIONS: Purification, spirituality, divination, alignment, inspiration

PLANETARY RULER: Moon

ELEMENTAL RULER: Water

DESCRIPTION: Sandalwood is a fragrant tree originating in India. In its native land, entire temples were built from sandalwood that are said to still emit its holy fragrance. To make Sandalwood essential oil, mature trees must be harvested and the heartwood steam distilled. Due to increased demand, Indian sandalwood has become threatened and extremely difficult and costly to obtain. However, both *S. album* and *S. spicatum* are now grown sustainably in Australia, and *S. paniculatum* (after a rough and storied history) is now grown sustainably in Hawaii. These will all serve well for magical and aromatherapeutic purposes.

MAGICAL USES: Sandalwood is primarily used in magic for purposes of purification and spiritual alignment. It is a key ingredient in spells for cleansing and protection such as Sacred Space Spray, Roll-On Energy Shield, and No More Nightmares Pillow Spray. It can be used to connect with the divine and receive messages from the spirit plane. As such, Sandalwood is called for in many preparations for divinatory work, including Intuition Roller, Third Eye Anointing Oil, and Soothsayer's Soak. Besides promoting spiritual alignment, the aroma of Sandalwood is thought by many to have aphrodisiac properties, justifying its inclusion in love spells like Anahata Opening and Aphrodite's Bath. Work with precious Sandalwood to attract wealth in alignment with spells and potions like Let the Good Times Roll and Straw into Gold Hair Oil.

OTHER USES: Sandalwood is often included in skincare and other health preparations.

PRECAUTIONS: None known, but source carefully and dilute appropriately.

BLENDS WELL WITH: Bergamot, Black Pepper, Black Spruce, Cassia, Cedarwood, Chamomile, Cinnamon, Clary Sage, Frankincense, Geranium, Grapefruit, Jasmine, Juniper, Lavender, Myrrh, Neroli, Nutmeg, Palmarosa, Patchouli, Rose, Tangerine, Vetiver, Ylang Ylang

SUBSTITUTE WITH: Frankincense, Palo Santo

Spearmint

COMMON NAME: Mint

LATIN NAME: *Mentha spicata*

FOLK NAME: Minthe, menthe, garden mint, lamb mint

POLARITY: Feminine

MAGICAL INTENTIONS: Healing, purification, prosperity, abundance

PLANETARY RULERS: Venus, Mercury

ELEMENTAL RULERS: Water, air

DESCRIPTION: Spearmint is essentially a gentler version of peppermint. In fact, it is one of the mints that peppermint was bred from. The discovery of a fourth-century Egyptian recipe for toothpaste containing mint is a testament to the fact that it has long been valued for its refreshing qualities. It grows abundantly and has numerous applications for health, wellness, and, of course, magic. The essential oil is steam distilled from the leaves.

MAGICAL USES: Mint's green and abundant nature make it a natural choice in money magic, and although mint the plant and mint the money-printing facility have separate etymologies, the coincidence cannot be ignored by practitioners of sympathetic magic. As such, you'll find Spearmint called for in spells such as Minting Money and Make It Rain. Its cleansing and purifying properties would make Spearmint a welcome addition to spells like Clear the Air or Going Away Party. Spearmint is also considered a healing herb. It is a key ingredient in the Happy Tummy Roller and Moontime Roller, and would make a fine addition to Miracle Massage Oil.

OTHER USES: Spearmint is often used for digestive support, to ease occasional discomfort, to support women's health, and to freshen breath.

PRECAUTIONS: Possible skin sensitivity; dilute appropriately.

BLENDS WELL WITH: Basil, Bergamot, Black Spruce, Chamomile, Citronella, Clary Sage, Eucalyptus, Geranium, Ginger, Grapefruit, Jasmine, Juniper, Lavender, Lemon, Lemongrass, Neroli, Orange, Peppermint, Petitgrain, Rose, Tangerine, Ylang Ylang

SUBSTITUTE WITH: Chamomile, Dill, Fennel, Ginger, Peppermint, Rosemary

Vetiver

COMMON NAME: Khus

LATIN NAME: *Chrysopogon zizanioides*

POLARITY: Feminine

MAGICAL INTENTIONS: Peace, relaxation, prosperity, protection

PLANETARY RULER: Venus

ELEMENTAL RULER: Earth

DESCRIPTION: Vetiver is a strong, earthy, and slightly sweet-smelling grass native to India. The essential oil is steam distilled from the roots, which grow deep down into the earth (as opposed to the more horizontal root systems of many other grasses), making it useful for erosion control. The stability it offers the earth may be applied in sympathetic magic for purposes of grounding, balancing, and protection. Vetiver grass is often made as an offering to Shiva and Ganesha. The smell is strong, and the consistency of Vetiver oil is so thick that it requires either a dropper or pipette or the patience of a bodhisattva to portion out. Perhaps I could stand the lesson in patience, but I have personally opted to fit my bottle of Vetiver with a dropper top.

MAGICAL USES: Vetiver's grounding and soothing properties make it useful in magical preparations such as Rest and Recover Roller and Soothing Soak. These same grounding and relaxing properties combined with its association with the earth element and earth magic make Vetiver appropriate for many types of wealth and prosperity magic, including such spells as Let the Good Times Roll and Good Fortune Fizz. It would not be out of place in magic for protecting personal property, or for achieving the appropriate state of focused relaxation necessary for divination. Vetiver is also appropriate for working with your ancestors and tapping into your roots.

OTHER USES: Vetiver is sometimes used in skincare, for grounding, to aid focus, to support women's health, and for sleep support. It is also popular as a fixative in the perfume industry.

PRECAUTIONS: Possible skin sensitivity; dilute appropriately. Avoid use during pregnancy.

BLENDS WELL WITH: Basil, Bergamot, Black Spruce, Cardamom, Cedarwood, Citronella, Clary Sage, Frankincense, Geranium, Grapefruit, Jasmine, Lavender, Lemon, Lemongrass, Lime, Myrrh, Neroli, Orange, Palmarosa, Patchouli, Rose, Sandalwood, Tangerine, Ylang Ylang

SUBSTITUTE WITH: Myrrh, Palo Santo, Patchouli, Sandalwood

Ylang Ylang

COMMON NAME: Cananga tree, perfume tree

LATIN NAME: *Cananga odorata*

POLARITY: Feminine

MAGICAL INTENTIONS: Love, lust, joy, peace, calming, creativity

PLANETARY RULER: Venus

ELEMENTAL RULER: Water

DESCRIPTION: The name "ylang ylang" comes from the Tagalog word for "wilderness," although it is commonly mistranslated as "flower of flowers," and it is easy to see why. The yellow star-shaped flowers of the cananga tree look like something out of a fairy tale, and their sweet, fruity-floral smell is just as enchanting. This evergreen tree is native to tropical Asia, and the essential oil is steam distilled from the flowers. Traditionally, the flowers are spread over the beds of newlywed couples in Indonesia, where they are thought to have aphrodisiac qualities.

MAGICAL USES: Ylang Ylang's associations with love, lust, and romance cannot be ignored. It is a key ingredient in several love spells in this book, including Anahata Opening, In the Mood for Love, and Aphrodite's Bath. Its aroma can be both uplifting and relaxing, which is one of the reasons you'll find it called for in the healing preparation Moontime Roller. Add Ylang Ylang to your personal perfumes and diffuser blends to invite a stimulating, uplifting, and loving energy into your body, your home, and your life.

OTHER USES: Ylang Ylang is frequently used for mood support, in skincare and haircare, and in the bedroom, in addition to its use in perfumery. It may also be used to support women's health.

PRECAUTIONS: Possible skin sensitivity; dilute appropriately.

BLENDS WELL WITH: Bergamot, Black Pepper, Cardamom, Cedarwood, Clove, Eucalyptus, Frankincense, Ginger, Grapefruit, Jasmine, Juniper, Lavender, Lemon, Lime, Orange, Neroli, Palmarosa, Patchouli, Peppermint, Petitgrain, Rose, Sandalwood, Tangerine, Vetiver

SUBSTITUTE WITH: Geranium, Jasmine, Neroli, Rose

PART IV

IN THIS PART, all the oil magic theory we've discussed thus far will come to life! The next five chapters comprise a collection of spells, charms, and rituals to get you started practicing the art of oil magic. Every oil has been included for a reason and the given blends have been concocted with care, but nothing is set in stone and thoughtful substitutions can be just as magically effective and aromatically pleasing. Refer to the Substitutions Chart and the oil profiles in chapter 6 for substitution suggestions if you are so inclined.

The following chapters include a selection of spells and potions for cleansing and protection, love and romance, wellness and healing, wealth and prosperity, and intuition and divination. Perform them as written, adapt them to your own practice, or use them as inspiration to write your own. However you may use them, they are here to guide and support you as you make every day magical and make magic every day.

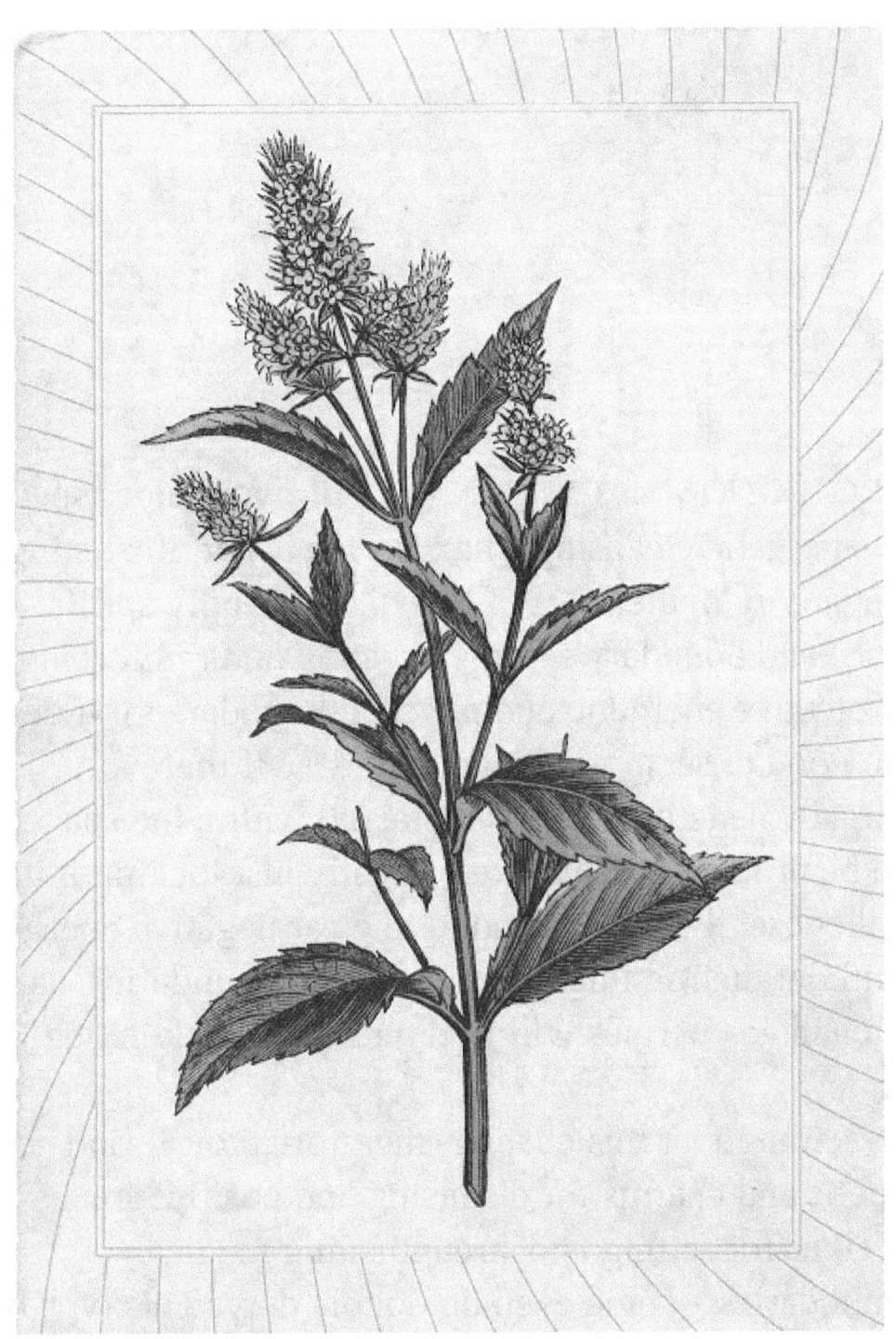

CHAPTER 7

Protection

PROTECTION MAGIC CONSISTS of two major aspects—energetic cleansing (the clearing away of existing negativity in the form of bad qi, unfriendly spirits, etc.) and boundary setting (creating and reinforcing protective energetic and physical boundaries). It does no good to set a protective boundary if there is already negative energy contained within the space to be protected, as you're basically just locking it in. Likewise, it does little good to clear negative energy without then setting and reinforcing boundaries, as unwanted energies will find their way back in due time.

Throughout this chapter, therefore, you'll find spells and charms for cleansing and purification as well as for setting and strengthening magical boundaries—some even do double duty. This type of magic forms a foundation for all other types of magic, as cleansing and protecting your energy and your space are key to fostering fertile ground for your intentions to manifest.

SIMPLE MAGIC

MAGIC ON THE GO

Mix Black Pepper and Clove to make a magical protective spray. Spray it on your doorstep or threshold to attract warmth and keep unwanted energies and visitors away.

Drip two or three drops each of Eucalyptus and Peppermint in the corner of your shower. The vapors will help clear the air and purify your energy from all negativity.

Add drops of Myrrh, Patchouli, or Rose to your body lotion or hair oil for a full-body energy shield that doubles as an entrancing perfume.

Diffuse Lavender, Rosemary, and Patchouli to create a peaceful atmosphere and purify the energy of anyone around.

Scent an aromatherapy inhaler with a drop of Rose and smell it anywhere to strengthen your heart chakra, fortify your boundaries, and raise your vibration.

Add your favorite cleansing and protective oils to your household cleaners to give them a magical boost.

Roll-On Energy Shield

Toss this in your bag and protect your energy wherever you go, no matter who's around. Optionally, you can add polished chips of black obsidian or a dried rosebud to the bottle before topping it off.

15 drops Myrrh

9 drops Sandalwood

3 drops Geranium

1 (10-milliliter) glass roller bottle

10 milliliters carrier oil

1. Combine the Myrrh, Sandalwood, and Geranium essential oils in the glass roller bottle and swirl gently to mix.
2. Inhale the synergy and visualize a white light filling your body and aura. The light acts as a shield, deflecting or burning away all unwanted subtle energy. Know that with this blend, you can call upon this light at any time.
3. Dilute with the carrier oil and assemble the bottle.
4. Roll onto your wrists and inner forearms to reinforce your energetic protection, visualizing the light shield as before. For extra oomph, roll it on in the shape of the rune Elhaz (ᛉ) and say, *I am protected*, or *I am divinely protected*.

Sacred Space Spray

Spray to hallow your space. This can be done instead of or in addition to circle casting. Alternatively, drop this blend in the diffuser—add just the oils to a dropper bottle to make a Sacred Space diffuser bomb.

15 drops Sage

10 drops Black Spruce

5 drops Palo Santo or 10 drops Sandalwood

4 drops Bergamot

3 drops Lavender

2 drops Cassia

1 (2-ounce) amber glass spray bottle

2 milliliters polysorbate 20 or 15 milliliters Everclear (emulsifier)

2 ounces distilled water

Smoky quartz chips (optional)

1. Combine the Sage, Black Spruce, Palo Santo, Bergamot, Lavender, and Cassia essential oils in the glass spray bottle and swirl gently to mix. Add the emulsifier, water, and smoky quartz chips (if using). Swirl to mix.

2. Spray throughout the desired area and say, *The air is clear, the space is sacred, by elements four now consecrated.*

3. Visualize a white light burning away all unwanted energy as you spray. Breathing deeply, walk through the mist you sprayed and see this same light cleansing and protecting you.

Clear the Air

To clear the air of stagnant energy, whip up this blend and get your diffuser going! To do a full home clearing, run the diffuser for a half hour in one area and then move it to a new location, repeating until your entire home feels renewed. For bonus points, take some time to clear clutter and organize your space while this blend clears the air. You can also use this opportunity to cleanse the energy of crystals and other objects in the diffuser mist.

180-milliliter diffuser

Distilled water

5 drops Citronella

2 drops Rosemary

2 drops Lavender

2 drops Black Spruce

---

1. Fill the diffuser with the water and add the Citronella, Rosemary, Lavender, and Black Spruce essential oils.
2. Start the diffuser and say, *In every corner of the room, drive out darkness, drive out gloom. Space be cleansed and air be clear, only good vibes welcome here!*
3. Feel the room's energy lifted and purified.

Protection Polish

This can be made with or without Rose. With, it seems to raise one's vibration and invoke the protection of the divine, or ascended, feminine; without, it is extremely grounding and energetically fortifying.

Glass mixing bowl

1 cup brown sugar

¼ cup sea salt

¼ cup carrier oil

¼ cup Castile soap

10 drops Myrrh

5 drops Patchouli

5 drops Frankincense

1 drop Rose (optional)

Airtight glass jar

1. In the glass mixing bowl, combine the brown sugar, sea salt, carrier oil, Castile soap, Myrrh, Patchouli, Frankincense, and Rose (if using) essential oils and transfer to the glass jar for storage in a cool, dry place.
2. With clean hands, portion out the desired amount before showering.
3. Use the body polish in the shower to scrub your body. As it exfoliates, visualize the salt, water, and Frankincense cleansing and purifying your energy. As it moisturizes, visualize the other oils

creating a protective barrier all over the surface of your body and expanding to include your aura.

Note: if this polish makes your shower slippery, add more Castile soap.

Death's Own Cloak

This recipe is inspired by a tale of four thieves who are said to have protected themselves from the Black Death with a botanical concoction. After looting the homes of many dead and dying with impunity, they were finally caught and their sentence lessened in exchange for their recipe.

Another tale inspired this recipe's name. It is a fable of three brothers who cheated death with magic, one of whom went on to live a long and happy life insured by death's own cloak of invisibility. This roller may not actually hide you from death itself, but still combines immune-supporting oils and defensive magic to great effect.

This recipe is for a 15-milliliter roller; if using 10-milliliter bottles, double the recipe and make three rollers for proper dilution.

---

6 drops Clove

6 drops Eucalyptus

6 drops Rosemary

3 drops Lemon

3 drops Tea Tree

1 drop Cassia

1 (15-milliliter) glass roller bottle

15 milliliters carrier oil

---

1. Combine the Clove, Eucalyptus, Rosemary, Lemon, Tea Tree, and Cassia essential oils in the glass roller bottle and swirl gently to mix.

2. Inhale the synergy, visualizing a black cloak surrounding and protecting you, dissolving anything that would cause harm.

3. Dilute with the carrier oil and assemble the bottle.

4. Repeat the visualization and apply the roller to your feet and spine when you desire extra magical protection and immune support.

No More Nightmares Pillow Spray

Spray this on your pillow each night before bed to promote restful sleep and defend against unpleasant dreams. For extra enchantment, add amethyst, smoky quartz, or obsidian chips.

15 drops Sandalwood

10 drops Lavender

10 drops Tangerine

5 drops Roman Chamomile

1 (2-ounce) glass spray bottle, blue or amber

2 milliliters polysorbate 20 or 15 milliliters Everclear (emulsifier)

2 ounces distilled water

Amethyst, smoky quartz, or obsidian chips (optional)

1. Combine the Sandalwood, Lavender, Tangerine, and Roman Chamomile essential oils in the glass spray bottle and swirl gently to mix.
2. Inhale the synergy and visualize a net of light surrounding your sleeping body in bed. Hold the vision and say, *As I lie asleep in bed, only sweet dreams fill my head.*
3. Add the emulsifier, water, and gem chips (if using). Swirl to mix.
4. Spray your pillow and the air above your bed, and repeat the visualization and incantation from step 2 before bed each night. Sweet dreams!

Front Door Defense

Your front door is your first line of defense in your home—yes, even against unwanted energy! Hang this charm on your door to help make sure the good stuff gets in and the bad stuff stays out.

Symbol of protection (see step 1)

9 drops Geranium

6 drops Black Pepper

3 drops Lemon

1 (2-milliliter) glass dropper bottle

1 milliliter carrier oil

Hanging hardware for door

1. Procure or create a decorative hanging that features a symbol of protection that is meaningful to you (e.g., a pentacle, goddess, protective runes, the hamsa, evil eye, etc.) and is made from a natural porous material such as untreated wood, unglazed ceramic, natural fiber cloth, or salt dough (see here).
2. Combine the Geranium, Black Pepper, and Lemon essential oils in the glass dropper bottle and swirl gently to mix.
3. Inhale the synergy and visualize warmth, joy, love, and positive feelings filling your home (or the space guarded by the door in question) and raising the space to a vibration that is incompatible with any unwanted energies that may approach from outside.

4. Hold the vision as you dilute the oils with the carrier oil, swirl, and massage some of the mixture into the symbol you chose. Hang the symbol on or near the door and periodically repeat the anointing and visualization as needed.

Four Corners Fortification

Your home is your castle, right? Make it a fortress with this spell, which employs four identical charm bags like magical turrets to protect a chosen space.

4 (4-inch) squares natural fiber black cloth

4 teaspoons salt, divided

4 drops Myrrh

4 drops Clove

4 drops Black Pepper

4 drops Geranium

4 small protective crystals (optional)

Twine or ribbon

1. Lay out the squares of cloth and spoon 1 teaspoon of salt into the center of each square. Drip 1 drop each of Myrrh, Clove, Black Pepper, and Geranium essential oils onto each mound of salt.

2. Place 1 small protective crystal (if using; four of the same, such as black obsidian, black tourmaline, or tiger's eye) in the center of each salt mound.

3. Gather the corners and tie the charm bags shut with the twine or ribbon.

4. Place each pouch in a corner of the chosen space. Using your finger, draw a golden thread of light in your mind's eye connecting each

charm bag to the next. Return to the start and see the golden thread completely surrounding the space.

5. As you see it in your mind's eye, say, *Four black corners mark the borders, evil OUT, witch's orders. The boundary now is fortified, safe is all that lies inside.*

Auric Protection Pendant

Wear this charm for an extra layer of energetic protection around your whole aura wherever you go. This charm is best created beneath a full moon, but any amount of moonlight is better than none.

3 drops Black Pepper

3 drops Myrrh

3 drops Geranium

1 drop Rose (optional)

1 drop Clove

1 (2-milliliter) clear glass dropper bottle

1 rose thorn

1 milliliter carrier oil

Small black pouch (optional)

Oil keeper or passive diffuser necklace

1. By moonlight, combine the Black Pepper, Myrrh, Geranium, Rose (if using), and Clove essential oils in the glass dropper bottle and say, *Pepper like fire to warm and defend, Myrrh to empower this protective blend, Geranium [and Rose] so love's power will stay, and Clove to keep negativity at bay.*

2. Add the thorn to the bottle, and say, *Light of moon and thorn of rose, shield my aura wherever I go.*

3. Cap the bottle and leave it to charge for a few hours in the moonlight. Before sunrise, dilute with the carrier oil and place in a small black

pouch (if using) or other dark place for safekeeping.

4. As needed, wear the necklace and fill or scent it with the oil blend. Visualize a protective barrier of rose vines and moonlight all around you and say, *By moonlight, clove, and peppercorn, by gentle flower and prickly thorn, I am protected, foes be warned.* Then boldly continue about your business.

Going Away Party

Do you sense that your home is infested with stubborn spirits? While it may sound unconventional, a friendly goodbye party for the spirits can work better and faster than forcing them out with sheer willpower and aggression.

Festive music

Festive attire

15 drops Frankincense

15 drops Myrrh

5 drops Cassia

5 drops Sage

2 milliliters polysorbate 20 or 15 milliliters Everclear (emulsifier)

2 ounces distilled water

1 (2-ounce) glass spray bottle

Gold coin (for safe passage to the other side)

1. Put on your music of choice and dress for a party! Raising the vibration in the space is an important first step.
2. Throughout the next steps, be sure to talk to your disembodied houseguest. Recount the memories you've shared, thank them for lessons learned, explain why they don't belong here, and share how excited you are for their homecoming.
3. Assemble the spell spray by combining the Frankincense, Myrrh, Cassia, and Sage essential oils, the emulsifier, and the water in the

glass spray bottle. Shake well to mix.

4. Starting in the farthest corners and working toward the exit, spray the entire home with the spell spray. This will encourage the spirit to move toward the exit.

5. As you spray, chant, *No more shall you haunt and wander and roam, for today is your happy journey home!* or something similar. At the exit, say goodbye, wish the spirit safe travels, and throw the coin out the door. Wave farewell, spray the doorway, shut the door, and turn off the music. The party is over.

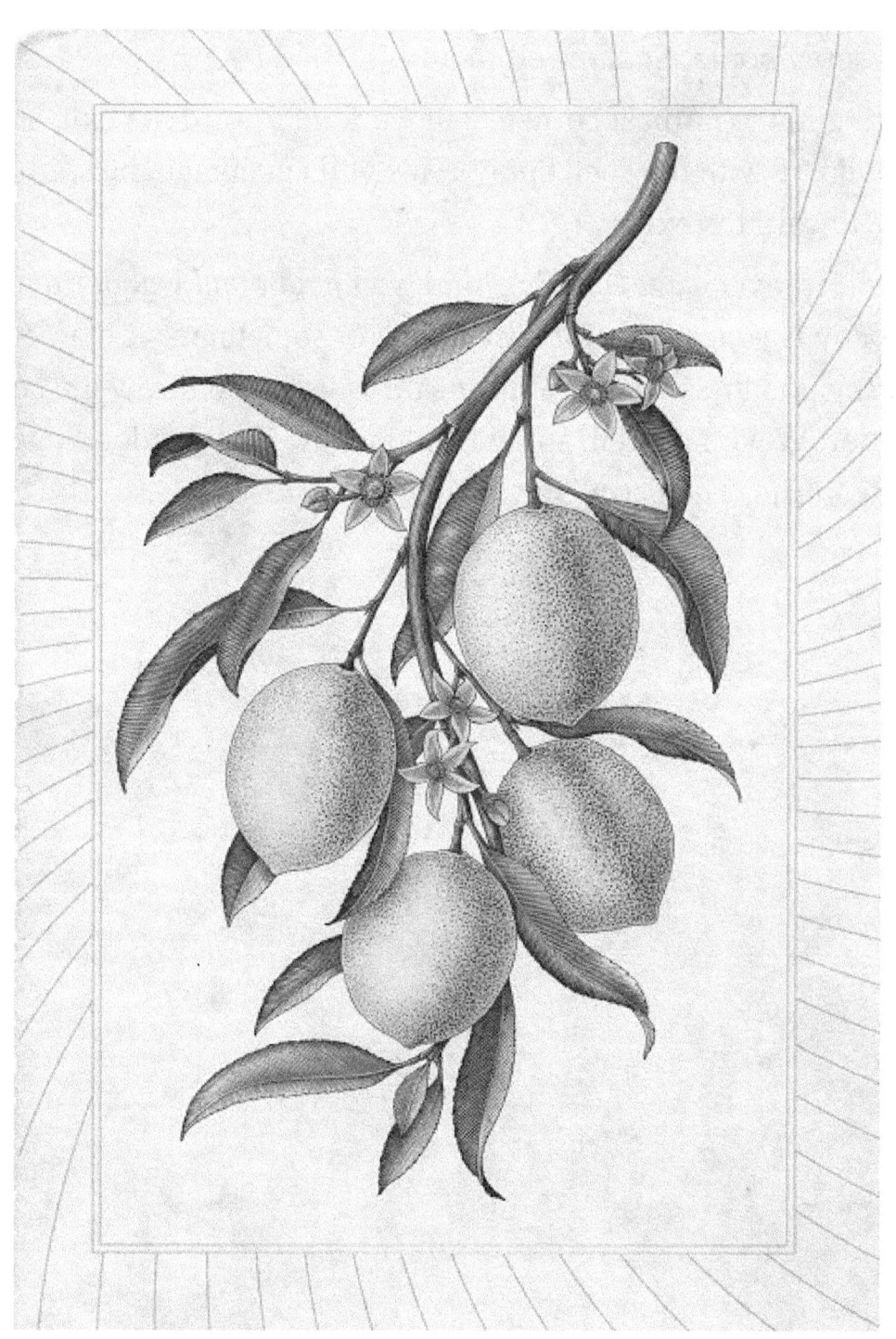

CHAPTER 8

Love

THE FIRST RULE of love magic is that we attract what we are ready for and believe we deserve. This means that self-love is a vital prerequisite for magically bringing more love into your life! You don't have to love yourself to *be* loved, but you *do* have to love yourself to intentionally *attract* the kind of love your heart yearns for. The principle of sympathetic magic is key here, too—that like attracts like and qi attracts more of the same. When you take time to love yourself (love is a verb) and have fun doing it, not only does your light shine brighter, but the universe picks up on how fun it is to love you and sends you more love.

This chapter begins with spells for self-love and moves on to self-care recipes infused with oils that energetically attract love and romance. Romance yourself, use your magic to give love to others, and soon you'll find yourself on the receiving end of more love than you'll know what to do with.

SIMPLE MAGIC

MAGIC ON THE GO

Remind yourself that you are worthy of love and care by taking time for yourself throughout the day to roll on your favorite oils and be present.

Write a love letter to yourself and scent the paper with a drop of your favorite flower oil. Read it whenever you need a reminder of just how lovable you are.

Write a love letter to someone and scent the paper with a drop of Cardamom, Nutmeg, or your favorite flower oil. Then, wear that oil next time you see them.

If you work with spirits or deities, leave an offering of a sugar cube with drops of Ginger and Cardamom with a petition for the love you seek.

Place one drop each of Frankincense, Rosemary, and Cardamom on a cotton ball and slip it under your pillow before bed to dream of your lover.

Self-Love Mirror Spell

Mirror work with affirmations and oils is a great way to go about cultivating the belief that you're worthy of love. When choosing an affirmation for this spell, it should be something you know to be true, although you might not always *feel* like it's true. The spell won't work if you *feel* like you're lying to yourself, but the point is to stretch the limits of your deepest beliefs about love.

Pen

Sticky note

Mirror (hands-free)

Dry-erase marker (optional)

3 drops Lavender

3 drops Orange

1 drop Geranium (optional)

Aromatherapy inhaler

1. Choose an affirmation. Write or find your own, or use one of these:
    - *It is safe for me to love and be loved.*
    - *I am worthy and deserving of love and affection.*
    - *I am learning to love myself more every day.*
2. Using a pen, write your chosen affirmation on a sticky note placed on your mirror. Alternatively, write with a dry-erase marker directly on your mirror.

3. Put the Lavender, Orange, and Geranium (if using) essential oils on the wick of an aromatherapy inhaler.

4. At least once a day, face the mirror and look yourself in the eye. Take a few deep breaths from the inhaler to ground yourself. Then, inhale the oils deeply and say the affirmation out loud on the exhale at least three times.

5. Do this as long and as often as you need to. Carry the inhaler with you so you can practice affirmations and deep breathing with or without a mirror whenever you find yourself slipping into old thought patterns.

6. When you have fully integrated the belief of your chosen affirmation into your life, choose another affirmation that stretches your beliefs about love and worthiness even further, and continue the practice.

Anahata Opening

Carry this solid perfume with you so you'll always be ready to tune in to, open, and align your heart chakra, no matter what annoyances life throws at you. When you raise yourself to love's vibration, love cannot help but find you.

This recipe makes 1 ounce. Keep the jackpot or share the love by splitting it into several smaller jars or compacts to give away.

---

1 tablespoon carrier oil

Double boiler

1 tablespoon beeswax

10 drops Lavender

10 drops Sandalwood

7 drops Ylang Ylang

3 drops Rose

1 (1-ounce) glass or metal container or several smaller ones to share the love

---

1. Put the carrier oil in the double boiler over medium-low heat. Add the beeswax and let it melt into the oil. Add the Lavender, Sandalwood, Ylang Ylang, and Rose essential oils, swirl to mix, and pour into the glass container. Let cool.

2. Whenever you notice yourself operating from a place of fear, judgment, or competition, anoint your heart chakra, third eye, throat, and behind your ears with this solid perfume and say, *I return to the energy of love. There is an infinite supply of love. I receive a*

reflection of what I give. Now, I choose to give love to myself and others.

Like a Moth to a Flame

When you shine your own inner light, you become more attractive, in every sense of the word. People and opportunities alike flock to brilliant spirits. Use this spell to amplify your inner light and attract love to you like a moth to a flame.

Note: This spell is *not* intended to manipulate a specific person; rather, it is intended to attract a particular energy to you.

Small knife (optional)

Beeswax chime candle and holder

Small glass bowl

¼ teaspoon carrier oil

1 drop Frankincense

1 drop Basil

1 drop Cardamom

1 drop Ginger

1 drop Rose, Geranium, or Ylang Ylang

---

1. Visualize the love or relationship you want to attract. It can be anything from a pen pal to a passionate romance to a life partner. Think about the kind of love and support you are looking for as well as the kind of love and support you like to give. Visualize the part of yourself that fits into this relationship glowing brighter and brighter, becoming a beacon to guide the love you desire toward you.

2. If using runes or sigils, use a knife to carve appropriate symbols into the candle. Alternatively, carve a word that represents the type of love you desire, such as "partnership," "passion," or simply "love."

3. In the bowl, combine the carrier oil with the Frankincense, Basil, Cardamom, Ginger, and Rose essential oils and dress the candle by coating it completely with the oil blend.

4. Light the candle and sit with it until it burns out. Spend this time visualizing yourself as the candle and your desire coming to you like a moth to a flame. You can also use this time to meditate, journal, or do a reading to clarify your next steps.

Yummy Love Scrub

The botanicals in this scrub are both purifying and heart-opening and are traditionally thought to have aphrodisiac properties. Merely indulging in a ritual this luxurious is an act of self-love and will make everything that happens afterward that much more deliciously smooth and sensual. For best results, follow up with Goddess Body Wash.

Large glass mixing bowl

1 cup brown sugar

¼ cup sea salt

¼ cup carrier oil

¼ cup Castile soap

10 drops Lavender

10 drops Geranium

10 drops Ylang Ylang

Airtight glass jar

1. In the mixing bowl, combine the sugar, salt, carrier oil, soap, and Lavender, Geranium, and Ylang Ylang essential oils, then transfer to the glass jar and store in a cool, dry place.

2. To use, with clean hands, portion out the desired amount for each shower. In the shower, give your body the gift of sweetness and flowers by scrubbing down every inch of your skin with this plant magic.

3. Emerge from the shower empowered with the magic of flowers, ready to receive and enjoy whatever sweetness life brings next.

Note: If this scrub makes your shower slippery, add more Castile soap.

Goddess Body Wash

Honey lends moisture and the magic of sweetness to this luxurious body wash that leaves store-bought suds feeling like wannabes. Patchouli and Rose make a classic combination for love and romance; save it for a special someone or make it your signature scent and invite love every day. While you could use an affirmation in tandem with this spell, it's best to lean into the sensual experience of washing your body with honey, patchouli, and the Queen of Flowers. For best results, use Yummy Love Scrub first and follow up with Goddess Body Wash in the shower.

⅓ cup honey

⅓ cup carrier oil

⅓ cup Castile soap

10 drops Patchouli

3 drops Rose

Glass pump bottle

1. Combine the honey, carrier oil, soap, and the Patchouli and Rose essential oils in the glass pump bottle and shake well to mix.
2. Lather, rinse, feel like a goddess or god of love, repeat.

In the Mood for Love

Fill the air with the scent of flowers and create an atmosphere that is ripe for romance with your trusty wingman or wingwoman—that is, your diffuser! Multiply the recipe and make a diffuser bomb beforehand to be ready to set the mood at the opportune moment. Good times to start the diffuser include right before the guest of honor arrives, immediately following dinner, or just as you get in the shower.

180-milliliter diffuser

Distilled water

3 drops Ylang Ylang

3 drops Tangerine

2 drops Clary Sage

1 drop Rose

1. Fill the diffuser with the water and add the Ylang Ylang, Tangerine, Clary Sage, and Rose essential oils.

2. Start the diffuser and say, *Love is all around me, this I know and believe. Magic of Love surrounds me, I am ready to give and receive!*

Lovers' Massage Oil

Keep this indulgent massage oil next to your bed and you'll always have a potion ready to help you and your lover get in the mood. Take turns and remember: Give love to receive love.

Note: Do be mindful where you put this on your body, as oils are not compatible with latex or polyisoprene and can degrade these materials.

20 drops Orange

10 drops Ginger

10 drops Cardamom

1 (4-ounce) glass bottle with pump or dropper top

4 ounces carrier oil

1. Combine the Orange, Ginger, and Cardamom essential oils in the glass bottle and swirl gently to mix.
2. Inhale the synergy and tune in to the energy of romantic stimulation and total relaxation.
3. Dilute with the carrier oil and assemble the bottle.
4. When the time is ripe, take turns giving and receiving massages with your lover. Find the joy in giving as well as receiving and allow yourself to relax completely into whatever happens next.

Love Potion No. 10

To stimulate the senses and support healthy circulation in all the right places, roll this romantic potion on your and your lover's inner thighs and lower belly before things get *too* steamy. Skip this if you're pregnant, though, or omit the Clary Sage.

   Note: Do be mindful where you roll this on your body, as oils are not compatible with latex or polyisoprene and can degrade these materials.

---

10 drops Orange

10 drops Ylang Ylang

5 drops Clary Sage

5 drops Cypress, Goldenrod, or Blue Spruce

2 drops Ginger

2 drops Nutmeg

1 drop Rose (optional)

1 (10-milliliter) glass roller bottle

10 milliliters carrier oil

---

1. Combine the Orange, Ylang Ylang, Clary Sage, Cypress, Ginger, Nutmeg, and Rose (if using) essential oils in the glass roller bottle and swirl gently to mix.

2. Inhale the synergy and tune in to the feeling of titillating romance and sensual excitement.

3. Dilute with the carrier oil and assemble the bottle.

4. When you're ready to turn up the heat, roll onto the inner thighs and below the navel to stimulate the body and ensnare the senses.

Freyja's Necklace

Norse mythology tells of a beautiful necklace belonging to the goddess Freyja that shone like fire and is thought to have added to her seductive power. It is that necklace, Brísingamen, that inspired this spell. Use any aromatherapy necklace that brings out your sensual side; it's even better if it is golden or contains amber in some form.

    Note: This charm is not intended to manipulate consent or bewitch a given target. It is merely intended to amplify and enhance your natural powers of attraction and seduction.

---

12 drops Sandalwood

10 drops Frankincense

10 drops Patchouli

5 drops Nutmeg

3 drops Rose

1 (5-milliliter) glass dropper bottle

3 milliliters grapeseed oil

Oil keeper or passive diffuser necklace

---

1. Combine the Sandalwood, Frankincense, Patchouli, Nutmeg, and Rose essential oils in the glass dropper bottle and swirl gently to mix.
2. Inhale the synergy and inhabit the feeling of irresistibility, the energy of attraction, the receptive space of seduction. Tune in to that feeling and remember it well.

3. Dilute with the grapeseed oil and swirl to mix. Fill an oil keeper pendant and apply to your neck and neckline as desired, or apply the blend to diffuser beads to wear. Repeat the visualization with each application as often as needed.

4. Let your magnetic personality shine!

Aphrodite's Bath

This recipe makes five standard-size bath bombs. You can use different essential oils than the ones listed here and add mica or dried flowers to customize this recipe to any intention (pink mica and roses are fun in this one, but totally optional). Save them for special occasions or use them to make any day special.

2 large glass mixing bowls

1 cup baking soda

½ cup cornstarch

½ cup Epsom salt

½ cup citric acid

3 tablespoons carrier oil

10 drops Ylang Ylang

10 drops Sandalwood

5 drops Tangerine

2 drops Rose

¾ tablespoon water

Bath bomb molds

1. In one large glass mixing bowl, combine the baking soda, cornstarch, Epsom salt, and citric acid.

2. In the second glass mixing bowl, combine the carrier oil, the Ylang Ylang, Sandalwood, Tangerine, and Rose essential oils, and the water.

3. Slowly add the dry ingredients to the wet ingredients. The mixture should hold its shape when squeezed. Pack tightly into the molds and let set for 1 to 2 minutes before unmolding. Let dry for 24 hours, then store in an airtight container.

4. When you're ready to use each bath bomb, you can make the bath extra special with rose quartz, mood lighting, and real roses, or just close your eyes and enjoy the aromas as you attune to the energy of love, romance, and receiving. To best prepare your body to soak up the magic, shower with Yummy Love Scrub and Goddess Body Wash before bathing.

5. Enter the water, submerge the bath bomb, and enjoy yourself! Soak up the magic of love and let yourself receive the joy of sensual experience.

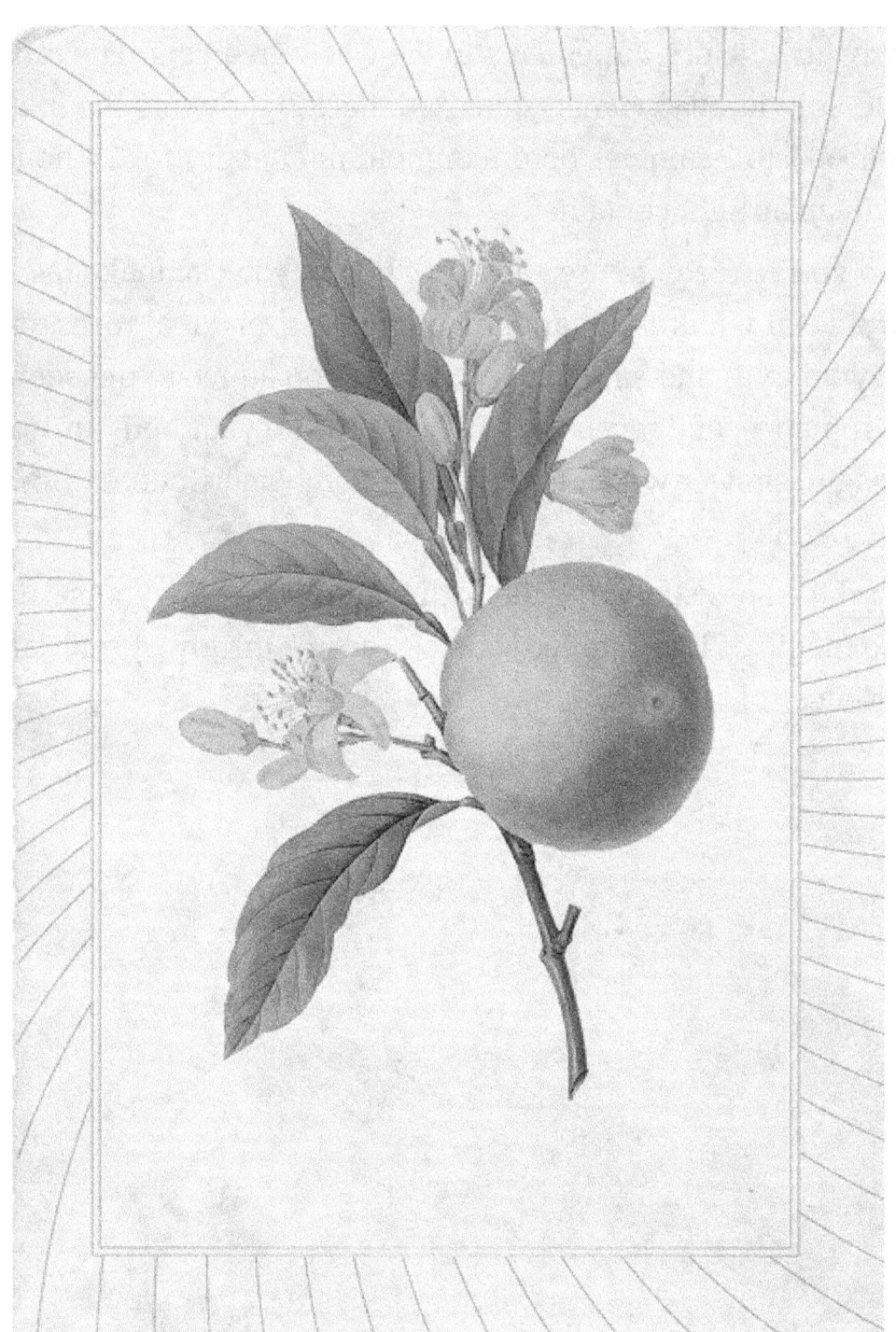

CHAPTER 9

Healing

HEALING MAGIC IS never meant to replace healthy habits or appropriate medical care. It can, however, assist with achieving wellness goals alongside these approaches. Many oils included in the spells throughout this chapter have been selected for healing properties that have historically been associated with them and their use. These properties, while traditionally accepted, have not been endorsed or evaluated by the FDA and, therefore, the spells and recipes in this chapter (and throughout the book) are for educational and entertainment purposes only.

All that said, our bodies are those of powerful magical creatures, and often will nonconsciously do (through automatic processes) what we consciously or subconsciously tell them to do. There are magical and mundane ways we can tell our bodies what to do, and the spells in this chapter take advantage of those methods—namely, olfactory memory, affirmation, and visualization. Incorporate these spells into your routine to support a healthy lifestyle and enjoy the miracle of magic while respecting its limits.

SIMPLE MAGIC

MAGIC ON THE GO

Mix a few drops of Frankincense into your lotion or moisturizer to keep your skin looking youthful and radiant.

Carve a candle with the name of a person who requires healing, and dress it with Helichrysum and Chamomile essential oils. Light the candle and visualize what ails them (or what ails you, if the spell is for you) melting away as the candle melts down.

Make a Lavender roller to have on hand for soothing occasional skin irritations, promoting restful sleep and relaxation, and easing occasional stress.

Diffuse three or four drops each of Lemon, Orange, and Peppermint to magically support motivation to exercise. During exercise, breathe deeply and say, I move my body with joy and ease.

Diffuse two or three drops each of Rosemary, Peppermint, Lemon, and Eucalyptus throughout your home to support a healthy immune system.

Just Breathe

The oils in this blend have historically been used to expand the breath and open the senses. Magically, their properties are balancing, soothing, uplifting, and healing. Turn to this spell whenever you need to *just breathe*.

180-milliliter diffuser

Distilled water

3 drops Eucalyptus

3 drops Lemon

3 drops Lavender

2 drops Peppermint

1. Fill the diffuser with the water and add the Eucalyptus, Lemon, Lavender, and Peppermint essential oils.
2. Start the diffuser and say between deep breaths, *Every breath is a healing breeze, I live my life with joy and ease.*

Soothing Salve

Keep a jar of this salve on hand to soothe and support your body in its natural healing process.

Double boiler

1 tablespoon beeswax

4 tablespoons coconut oil, solid

4 tablespoons olive oil

1 (4-ounce) airtight glass jar

20 drops Lavender

20 drops Frankincense

20 drops Helichrysum

10 drops Clary Sage

1. In the double boiler over medium-low heat, melt the beeswax and coconut oil with the olive oil. Stir to mix and visualize positive healing energy being incorporated into the oil.
2. Run the sealed glass jar under hot tap water to warm it in preparation for receiving the melted salve.
3. Combine the Lavender, Frankincense, Helichrysum, and Clary Sage essential oils in the glass jar.
4. Pour the melted oil mixture into the jar with the essential oils and visualize the positive healing energy filling the jar. You will have a tiny bit left over and can offer it to the earth as a token of gratitude for the earth's gifts of healing.

5. Let the mixture cool. When it has solidified, it is ready to use. To use, scoop up the desired amount with your fingers or a small spatula and apply to areas in need of soothing. Visualize the positive healing energy you stirred into the salve infusing your body as it soaks into your skin.

Inner Peace Inhaler

Inner peace is almost always just a few deep breaths away—you just have to make time for them! The oils in this blend are thought to have peaceful, calming, and uplifting magical properties. Call on this spell to soothe your spirit anytime you need to slow down.

4 drops Lavender

4 drops Orange

1 drop German Chamomile

Aromatherapy inhaler

1. Put the Lavender, Orange, and German Chamomile essential oils on the wick of an aromatherapy inhaler. As you do, attune to the energy of inner peace with slow, deep breaths and say out loud, *Lavender to soothe, Orange to uplift, Chamomile to calm, energy shift.*

2. Whenever you feel you could benefit from a moment of calm and a return to peace, pull out your Inner Peace Inhaler and take a few deep breaths. You can incorporate an affirmation if it helps you, but sometimes silence is the medicine our souls need; follow your intuition. On your deep breaths, try to make your exhales longer than your inhales. Do this as often as you need to.

Moontime Roller

This roller recipe is especially beneficial and soothing for people who experience a monthly cycle but can be used by anyone to magically assist with soothing and relaxing the body and mind. Skip this if you're pregnant, however, or omit the Clary Sage and cut the other oils in half. This roller especially benefits from being charged under the full moon if you are able to do so.

15 drops Lavender

10 drops Clary Sage

5 drops Ylang Ylang

5 drops Spearmint

1 (10-milliliter) glass roller bottle

Amethyst chips (optional)

10 milliliters carrier oil

1. Combine the Lavender, Clary Sage, Ylang Ylang, and Spearmint essential oils in the glass roller bottle and swirl gently to mix. Add a few amethyst chips (if using).
2. Dilute with the carrier oil and assemble the bottle. Swirl to mix and visualize soothing and healing positive qi being swirled into the oils.
3. When you need the soothing magic of the Moontime Roller, roll it on your lower belly, inner wrists, and lower back, breathing in the soothing and healing positive qi you previously infused into the oils.

Wash Your Worries Away

If afternoon naps in the sun were a body wash, this would be it. Use this body wash all over to infuse your whole self with soothing Lavender, fragrant Frankincense, and uplifting Orange. From avocado to Orange, each ingredient magically supports the natural healing processes of your body and mind. Be sure to store this safely in the shower so it will not fall and break.

⅓ cup avocado oil

⅓ cup Castile soap

⅓ cup honey

40 drops Lavender

40 drops Frankincense

20 drops Orange

Glass pump bottle

1. Combine the avocado oil, soap, honey, and the Lavender, Frankincense, and Orange essential oils in the glass pump bottle and shake well to mix.
2. With your hands on the bottle, visualize rays of golden sunlight and a cloud of butterflies blessing the body wash with peaceful, healing, and uplifting energy.
3. To use, visualize the sunlight and butterflies coming out of the bottle as you pump the body wash into your hands. Lather, rinse, feel yourself filled with joy and peace, repeat.

Soothing Soak

This recipe makes five standard-size bath bombs. These are great to have on hand for the end of the workweek, or whenever you need to soak away your worries, put your cares on a shelf, and float away on an ocean of repose.

2 large glass mixing bowls

1 cup baking soda

½ cup cornstarch

½ cup Epsom salt

½ cup citric acid

3 tablespoons carrier oil

10 drops Frankincense

10 drops Cedarwood

5 drops Vetiver

5 drops Lavender

¾ tablespoon water

Bath bomb molds

1. In one large glass mixing bowl, combine the baking soda, cornstarch, Epsom salt, and citric acid.
2. In the second glass mixing bowl, combine the carrier oil, the Frankincense, Cedarwood, Vetiver, and Lavender essential oils, and the water.

3. Slowly mix the dry ingredients into the wet ingredients. While mixing, visualize yourself folding in a golden light of positive healing energy. The mixture should hold its shape when squeezed. Pack tightly into the molds and let set for 1 to 2 minutes before unmolding. Let dry for 24 hours, then store in an airtight container.

4. When you're ready to use each bath bomb, prepare the environment to be as soothing and relaxing as possible. Make sure you have plenty of water to stay hydrated (and maybe a mug of tea on the side) and that you will not be disturbed. Play some peaceful music, and shower beforehand to be able to soak up as many good vibes as possible.

5. Enter the water, submerge the bath bomb, and enjoy yourself. Allow yourself to fully relax. Feel the water wash away your worries and cares, and infuse your body, mind, and spirit with deep healing energy.

Rest and Recover Roller

Sleep is one of the most important ways we can heal and take care of ourselves. Keep this roller by your bedside to support your body's rest and recovery during sleep.

5 drops Lavender

5 drops Cedarwood

5 drops Vetiver

2 drops Chamomile

1 (10-milliliter) glass roller bottle

Pipette (optional)

10 milliliters carrier oil

1. Combine the Lavender, Cedarwood, Vetiver, and Chamomile essential oils in the glass roller bottle and swirl gently to mix. (A pipette may be necessary for the Vetiver.)

2. Dilute with the carrier oil and assemble the bottle. Swirl to mix and visualize purple clouds of restorative sleep spiraling into the oil.

3. When you need a little magic to support your sleep, roll this blend onto your inner wrists, chest, and back of neck, and visualize the enchanting purple clouds you previously infused into the mixture permeating your skin and filling your mind. Sweet dreams!

Summon the Sandman

The Sandman is known throughout Western and Northern European folklore as a helpful figure who sprinkles magical sand into the eyes of those he visits, inspiring deep sleep and beautiful dreams. Diffuse this blend to summon magical assistance with entering the land of sleep and dreams.

180-milliliter diffuser

Distilled water

4 drops Cedarwood

4 drops Lavender

2 drops German Chamomile

1. Fill the diffuser with the water and add the Cedarwood, Lavender, and German Chamomile essential oils.

2. Start the diffuser and say after a few deep breaths, *By Cedar, Lavender, and Chamomile, Sandman, help me sleep awhile. Send me sleep on moonlight beams, and grant me only peaceful dreams.*

3. Then lie down, close your eyes, and focus only on your breathing until sleep takes you.

Miracle Massage Oil

This massage oil is great to have on hand for tired muscles after a demanding workout or a long day.

   Note: Wintergreen is the most important ingredient in this blend, but it *must* be 100 percent plant-derived and properly distilled. Many Wintergreens on the market, or "oil of wintergreen," are pure lab-synthesized ester (methyl salicylate), and while they may smell similar to or even the same as plant-derived wintergreen, the chemical structure is not the same. Consult a doctor before use if you are on any type of blood-thinning medication.

---

20 drops Wintergreen

20 drops Frankincense

10 drops Helichrysum

10 drops Peppermint

10 drops Clove

1 (4-ounce) glass bottle with pump or dropper top

4 ounces carrier oil

---

1. Combine the Wintergreen, Frankincense, Helichrysum, Peppermint, and Clove essential oils in the glass bottle and swirl gently to mix. Visualize a golden healing light being swirled into the mixture.
2. Dilute with the carrier oil and assemble the bottle.
3. After a long day, massage this blend into tired muscles such as those of the arms, legs, shoulders, hips, neck, and back. (Better yet, get a friend to lend a hand!) As you do so, visualize the golden healing

light you infused into the oils seeping into your skin and infusing your muscles with restorative energy. Note: Keep away from sensitive areas such as the face, armpits, genitals, and open wounds.

Happy Tummy Roller

Keep this roller around and you'll always have a little something to keep your tummy happy. Roll this on after heavy meals or anytime your tummy could use a little help from plant magic to stay settled and at peace.

5 drops Ginger

5 drops Cardamom

5 drops Fennel

5 drops Peppermint

5 drops Spearmint

1 (10-milliliter) glass roller bottle

10 milliliters carrier oil

1. Combine the Ginger, Cardamom, Fennel, Peppermint, and Spearmint essential oils in the glass roller bottle and swirl gently to mix.
2. Dilute with the carrier oil and assemble the bottle. Swirl to mix and visualize a golden healing light being incorporated into the oils.
3. When you need a little magic to keep your tummy happy and support your body's normal healthy digestive system, roll this potion in circles around your belly button and visualize the golden healing light entering your body to help keep everything balanced and moving along properly.

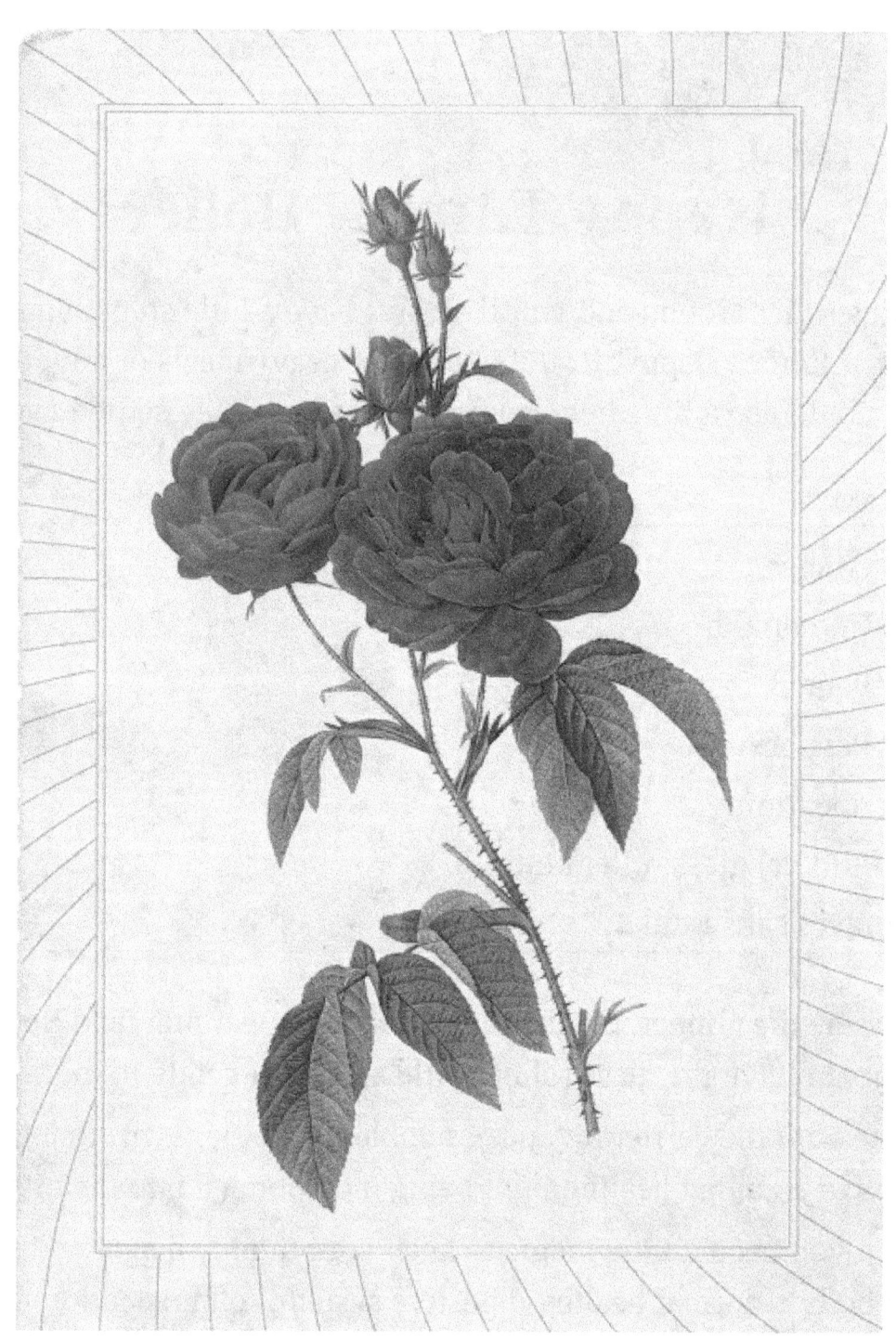

CHAPTER 10

Wealth

MAGIC FOR MANIFESTING wealth, prosperity, and abundance begins with your mindset. The spells in this chapter make use of the magic of plants and oils traditionally associated with prosperity and riches to cultivate an attitude of gratitude, a belief in abundance (as opposed to scarcity), and a feeling of luxury. With gratitude, you tell the universe what you appreciate and want more of and shift your perspective to immediate positive effect. Belief in abundance or having more than enough is called the abundance mindset and is necessary for attracting anything (especially wealth) into your life. Finally, giving yourself the sort of sensual experiences you associate with wealth and luxury allows you to start making those feelings your reality *now*.

SIMPLE MAGIC

MAGIC ON THE GO

Scent a cotton ball with a few drops of Spearmint and Ginger and stuff it in your piggy bank (or a similar container for keeping bills and coins) to magically encourage your savings to grow.

Coat a golden coin in honey mixed with a drop of Ginger and bury it beneath a fruit tree to encourage your wealth to "be fruitful and multiply."

Scent a cotton ball with essential oils of Black Pepper and Clove and keep it in your wallet to both attract wealth and ward against unwise spending and financial trouble.

Mix a few drops each of Basil and Orange oil into unscented liquid hand soap to encourage positive financial transactions whenever money changes hands.

Cover a $2 bill (or the largest bill you can afford not to spend) with drawings of abundant trees, leaves, flowers, and fruit, and scent it with Spearmint, Basil, Orange, and Frankincense. Keep it at the bottom of your wallet and never spend it.

Gratitude Journal

Gratitude for what we already have is one of the most important elements of attracting abundance. Create a scented gratitude journal and write in it daily to notice and attract more of what you have to be grateful for.

Journal

2 drops Orange

2 drops Patchouli

1 drop Ginger

1 drop Clove

1. Select a journal to be your gratitude and manifestation journal and mark it as such.
2. Drop the Orange, Patchouli, Ginger, and Clove essential oils onto the inside back cover of the journal.
3. Every day, or as often as possible, write down the things you are grateful for that day. You can keep it short and sweet or go into paragraphs of detail—whatever feels right to you.
4. You can also use this journal to write out your manifestations (things you are inviting and welcoming into your life), but write them in a present tense gratitude format. For example, if you have a very old car, or none at all, you can write, "I am so grateful to be saving up for my new car," or "I am so grateful to be welcoming a new car into my life."

5. Periodically revisit the things you have written to tune in to the gratitude you felt when you wrote them and remind yourself of how abundant and full your life already is.

Abundance Mindset Inhaler

So much of feeling and achieving abundance is our mindset, that is, our attitudes, perceptions, and perspective. Do you believe you have enough? Do you believe there is more than enough for everyone? A scarcity mindset says there is not enough for everyone to thrive, and we must compete. It motivates us to act from a place of fear—fear that if we don't do what it says, we won't have enough. An abundance mindset says there is always more than enough for everyone to thrive, and we must cooperate and collaborate to allocate resources where they are most needed. It motivates us to act from a place of empowered love, without fear. Turn to this spell to reinforce or return to an abundance mindset. From there, you can make all your decisions and live your entire life in that place of empowered love.

3 drops Orange

3 drops Patchouli

2 drops Cardamom

Aromatherapy inhaler

1. Put the Orange, Patchouli, and Cardamom essential oils on the wick of an aromatherapy inhaler. If you accidentally add extra drops, it's okay. Know that there is always more than enough.
2. Inhale from the wick and attune to the expansive energy of abundance. On each exhale, say out loud, *I am abundant always, in all ways.*

3. Whenever you notice you could benefit from a return to an abundance mindset, pull out this inhaler, take a few deep breaths, and repeat the affirmation (or another abundance affirmation of your choosing) as needed.

Pocket Pyrite

Keep this charm in your pocket or bag to attract the energy of wealth and abundance. Pyrite is ideal for this spell because of its golden appearance, association with wealth and prosperity, and because its structure usually includes little crystalline pockets for essential oil to seep into. This charm is designed for a pocket or bag, but can be adapted for a safe, piggy bank, or other container used for bills and coins.

9 drops Orange

8 drops Patchouli

8 drops Ginger

8 drops Clove

4 drops Cardamom

3 drops Myrrh

1 (2-milliliter) glass dropper bottle

Piece of pyrite, pocket-size

Small cloth bag or square

1. Combine the Orange, Patchouli, Ginger, Clove, Cardamom, and Myrrh essential oils in the glass dropper bottle and swirl gently to mix.
2. Inhale the synergy and take a moment to be grateful for all that you already have in your life, visualizing everything that you love and

value expanding and multiplying. Know that there is always more than enough.

3. Take the pyrite in your receiving (nondominant) hand and lay your dominant hand over it, holding the vision from step 2.

4. Using your dominant hand, apply 1 to 3 drops of the oil blend to crystalline cavities in the pyrite and, as you do, visualize the expansive energy of abundance from your vision filling the stone.

5. Say out loud, *By Orange and Patchouli, by Ginger, Cardamom, Myrrh, and Clove, my pocket is ever a treasure trove.*

6. To protect both the stone and your skin, place the stone in the small bag or wrap it in cloth, and then place it where you want it to work its magic. Every new moon, or whenever the smell fades, repeat steps 2 to 5.

Make It Rain

This joyful and refreshing blend incorporates some of the brighter scents of plants traditionally associated with money magic. Several of these "prosperity plants" are also associated with clear thinking and positivity in general. Diffuse this blend at the start of your day, in a place of business, or when making financial decisions.

180-milliliter diffuser

Distilled water

4 drops Orange

3 drops Spearmint

3 drops Peppermint

2 drops Basil

1. Fill the diffuser with the water and add the Orange, Spearmint, Peppermint, and Basil essential oils.
2. Start the diffuser and say, *Fruit of gold and leaves of green, magic make it rain on me; it's already started, it's already happening, abundance beyond my wildest imagining.*

Minting Money

It is often said that what you put out comes back to you. Because wealth and abundance are literally "more than enough," one of the best ways to encourage these things is to give them away. Money is just bits of paper and metal or numbers on a screen; what makes it valuable to you is that it can be exchanged for things you want and need. It derives its power from being spent—so spend it (wisely)! And when you do, send a little plant magic out with it.

---

15 drops Peppermint

15 drops Spearmint

10 drops Ginger

1 (2-ounce) glass spray bottle

2 milliliters polysorbate 20 or 15 milliliters Everclear (emulsifier)

2 ounces distilled water

Citrine or green aventurine chips (optional)

Cash money (bills or coins)

Towel

---

1. Combine the Peppermint, Spearmint, and Ginger essential oils in the glass spray bottle and swirl gently to mix. Add the emulsifier, water, and citrine chips (if using). Swirl to mix.
2. Lay out all the cash money you currently possess in a single layer on a towel, spray it all three times over, and say, *Three times three times three times three, every dollar I spend returns to me.* As you spray,

visualize the money in front of you growing and multiplying like a flourishing mint plant.

3. Let the money dry, return it to your wallet, and revisit this visualization anytime you spend money.

4. Whenever a new chunk of change or stack of bills comes into your possession, repeat steps 2 and 3.

Let the Good Times Roll

Stress is one of the biggest enemies of abundance. It is rooted in the idea that there is not enough time, not enough energy, or not enough money or resources to do what is necessary. When we release stress, we make way for the attitude of abundance. Use this roller spell to help you return to an abundance mindset, from which you can appreciate the gift of life and all it has to offer free of fear, because you know that the universe provides. Roll it on and let the good times roll!

10 drops Sandalwood

10 drops Vetiver

5 drops Orange

5 drops Lavender

1 (10-milliliter) glass roller bottle

Citrine chips (optional)

10 milliliters carrier oil

1. Combine the Sandalwood, Vetiver, Orange, and Lavender essential oils in the glass roller bottle and swirl gently to mix. Add a few citrine chips (if using).

2. Dilute with the carrier oil and assemble the bottle. Swirl to mix and visualize a harmonious and positive golden light being swirled into the oils.

3. Roll onto your inner wrists, clavicle, and back of neck as needed, and visualize the golden light you infused into the oils melting away your tension and stress as it seeps into your skin. As you do, say, *I let go of*

stress and surrender to the guidance of spirit, or another affirmation that resonates with you.

Liquid Gold Body Wash

One of the best ways to manifest abundance is to cultivate the *feeling* of abundance by treating yourself the way you would if you felt truly abundant. Much of magic is switching from the "when I feel X, I will do Y" mindset to the "when I do Y, I feel X" mindset (e.g., from "when I feel abundant, I will use really nice body wash" to "when I use really nice body wash, I feel abundant"). Lather up with this plant-magic equivalent of liquid gold to cultivate that feeling every day! Be sure to store this safely in the shower where it will not fall and break.

30 drops Orange

30 drops Frankincense

20 drops Patchouli

10 drops Myrrh

1 (10-ounce or larger) glass pump bottle

⅓ cup jojoba oil

⅓ cup Castile soap

⅓ cup honey

Gold mica or 24k gold flake (optional)

1. Combine the Orange, Frankincense, Patchouli, and Myrrh essential oils in the glass pump bottle and swirl gently to mix.
2. Inhale the synergy and attune to the expansive energy of abundance. Visualize the most abundant version of your life you can imagine.

3. Holding the vision, add the jojoba oil, Castile soap, honey, and mica (if using). Shake well to mix.

4. During each use, return to the vision of your most abundant life. Imagine that as you lather this potion over your body, you are gilding yourself with that vision of abundance. Lather, visualize, rinse, repeat.

Midas Touch Body Butter

Making your own bath and body products is very economical, and the results are incredibly luxurious. All it takes is a few simple ingredients and a little time to make this body butter that will have you feeling like a million bucks!

Double boiler

½ cup shea butter

Glass mixing bowl

Whisk

1½ teaspoons arrowroot powder

¼ cup grapeseed oil

20 drops Patchouli

20 drops Frankincense

20 drops Orange

5 drops Rose

Electric mixer

Widemouthed glass jar with a lid

1. In the double boiler over medium-low heat, melt the shea butter. Meanwhile, in the glass mixing bowl, whisk the arrowroot powder into the grapeseed oil. Then, combine the melted shea butter with the grapeseed oil mixture.

2. Add the Patchouli, Frankincense, Orange, and Rose essential oils to the mixture, then stir to combine, visualizing the liquid gold energy of

abundance itself being stirred into the mixture.

3. Let chill, covered, in the freezer for about 20 minutes.

4. Using the electric mixer, whip the mixture until it at least doubles in volume (if the mixture is too liquid to whip, chill longer; if too solid, melt again with the double boiler and chill for less time). Scoop into the glass jar and seal.

5. To use, scoop your desired amount with clean hands or a spoon and massage into your skin. Visualize the golden expansive energy of abundance seeping into your skin and feel like a million bucks!

Straw into Gold Hair Oil

This hair oil will nourish dry locks, enhancing the appearance of healthy, shining hair. Its scent will linger all day, making millers' sons and daughters smell and feel like royalty.

20 drops Sandalwood

10 drops Orange

10 drops Patchouli

5 drops Rose

1 (2-ounce) glass bottle with pump or dropper top

2 ounces jojoba oil

1. Combine the Sandalwood, Orange, Patchouli, and Rose essential oils in the glass bottle and swirl gently to mix.
2. Inhale the synergy and visualize all things "straw" in your life being spun into "gold" (i.e., anything in your life that you've "settled" for or that stimulates feelings of scarcity, lack, or fear being transformed into its most positive and abundant form).
3. Dilute with the jojoba oil, swirl, and assemble the bottle.
4. Each morning or after each shower, massage this blend into your hair by first rubbing your oiled hands together and then running them through your hair, focusing especially on the dry ends. As you do so, imagine that you are spinning straw into gold, both in your hair and in your life.

Good Fortune Fizz

This recipe makes five standard-size bath bombs—in other words, *more than enough*. Keep one or two for yourself and give the rest away, in true abundant fashion. After all, you can always make more.

2 large glass mixing bowls

1 cup baking soda

½ cup cornstarch

½ cup Epsom salt

½ cup citric acid

3 tablespoons carrier oil

10 drops Frankincense

10 drops Patchouli

10 drops Vetiver

5 drops Jasmine or Chamomile

¾ tablespoon water

1 teaspoon gold mica (optional)

Bath bomb molds

1. In one large glass mixing bowl, combine the baking soda, cornstarch, Epsom salt, and citric acid.
2. In the second glass mixing bowl, combine the carrier oil, the Frankincense, Patchouli, Vetiver, and Jasmine essential oils, the water, and the mica (if using).

3. Slowly mix the dry ingredients into the wet ingredients. While mixing, visualize yourself folding in a golden light of prosperity and good fortune. The mixture should hold its shape when squeezed. Pack tightly into the molds and let set for 1 to 2 minutes before unmolding. Let dry for 24 hours, then store in an airtight container.

4. When you're ready to use each bath bomb, prepare the environment to feel as luxurious as possible. Surround yourself with crystals, candles, coins, and symbols of prosperity (optional but recommended). Bring a favorite beverage and perhaps some fruit (apples, grapes, and oranges are all prosperity symbols).

5. Then, enter the water, submerge the bath bomb, and bathe in your good fortune. Allow yourself to fully relax and know that you are provided for. Feel the golden light of prosperity and good fortune permeating your skin and renewing your spirit. Know that life is good.

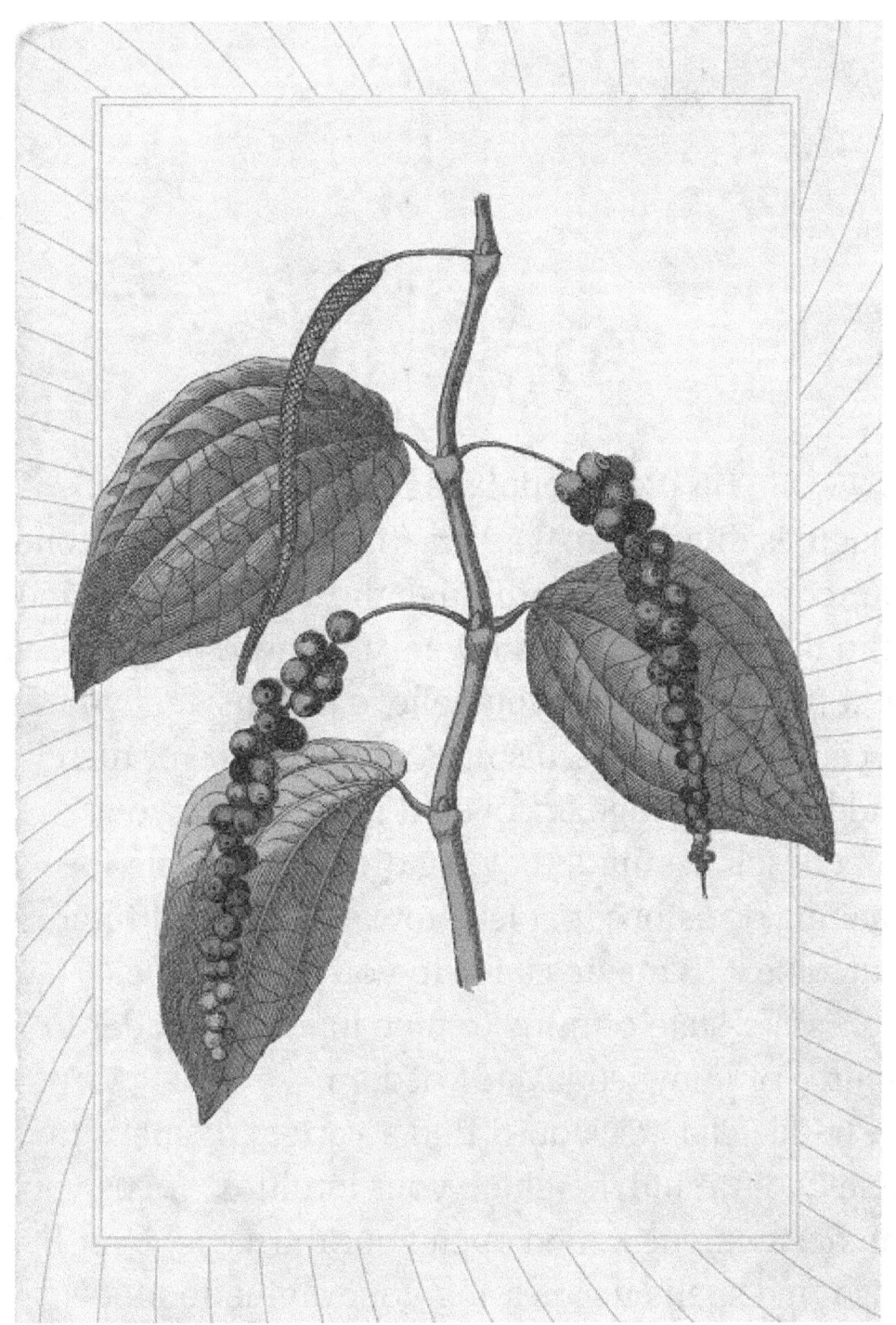

CHAPTER 11

Divination

ONE OF THE most popular and useful aspects of magic is divination: The practice of peering beyond our conscious minds, through the subconscious and into the unknown for answers about our past, present, and future. Whether you believe the answers you receive are gifts from spirits or the divine or merely hidden knowledge uncovered from within your subconscious mind, they are often invaluable for making decisions that lead toward a desired future outcome. Oil magic can help you achieve the necessary state of mind to tune in to this hidden source of knowledge and wisdom.

In this chapter, you'll find a variety of spells to relax your mind, heighten your intuition, focus your higher awareness, and open your third eye. You'll also find spells for blessing your divination tools, a guide to candle scrying with oils, and a tutorial for making your own oil-infused runes!

SIMPLE MAGIC

MAGIC ON THE GO

Scent a diffuser necklace with a third eye–opening oil such as Sandalwood and use it as a pendulum.

Diffuse Patchouli when attempting to communicate with the spirits of the dead.

Assign meanings to several of your oils based on possible answers to a question you have, and with closed eyes, mix them up and select one. Diffuse or wear that oil for the day while you act on the wisdom received.

Make a glass cleaner with two parts distilled water, one part white vinegar, and Rosemary, Lemon, Sandalwood, and Jasmine essential oils, and use it to clean bowls or mirrors for use in scrying.

Ask Spirit to guide you to what you need right now and pull three cards from a favorite tarot or oracle deck. Then, use those cards as inspiration to pick three oils for a custom blend based on their magical meanings and correspondences (you can use this book as a guide). For example, if you pull the Two of Cups, the Sun, and the Moon, you might make a blend of Geranium, Orange, and Jasmine.

Intuition Roller

Roll this on before pulling cards, reading tea leaves, or anytime your intuition could use an extra boost. You can also roll it around the perimeter of an altar cloth or casting cloth to enhance readings.

10 drops Sandalwood

10 drops Frankincense

5 drops Lavender

5 drops Rosemary

1 (10-milliliter) glass roller bottle

Amethyst chips (optional)

10 milliliters carrier oil

1. Combine the Sandalwood, Frankincense, Lavender, and Rosemary essential oils in the glass roller bottle and swirl gently to mix. Add a few amethyst chips (if using).

2. Dilute with the carrier oil and assemble the bottle. Swirl to mix and visualize the sparkling light of divine guidance being swirled into the oils.

3. Roll onto your inner wrists, ankles, heart, or back of neck as needed, and visualize the sparkling light you infused into the oils creating a channel or bridge of clear communication between you and Spirit. As you do, say, *I am connected to the divine and I am open to receiving guidance for my highest good and the highest good of all.*

Aura of Extrasensory Perception

Diffuse this blend to set the mood and enhance the space for divination, meditation, inner journeys, or any time you want to create an aura of enhanced awareness.

180-milliliter diffuser

Distilled water

4 drops Frankincense

4 drops Sandalwood

2 drops Black Spruce

2 drops Myrrh

1. Fill the diffuser with the water and add the Frankincense, Sandalwood, Black Spruce, and Myrrh essential oils.
2. Start the diffuser and say, *The Universe is always speaking to me, and I am always listening.*
3. Perform your divination nearby after the diffuser has permeated your senses and filled the space. You can even scry in the diffuser mist itself!

Third Eye Anointing Oil

This is one of those oils that is worth storing in a special fancy bottle, should you have one itching to be used. If not, a dropper bottle will work just fine. Keep it on your altar and apply it to your third eye before divination, meditation, ritual, or spellwork.

9 drops Frankincense

7 drops Sandalwood

5 drops Helichrysum

2 drops Jasmine

2 drops Rose

1 (15-milliliter) glass bottle with dropper top

15 milliliters carrier oil

1. Combine the Frankincense, Sandalwood, Helichrysum, Jasmine, and Rose essential oils in the glass bottle and swirl gently to mix.
2. Inhale the synergy and visualize your third eye wide open, with a beam of light connecting it to the heavens.
3. Dilute with the carrier oil, swirl, and assemble the bottle.
4. Before practicing divination, meditation, ritual, or spellwork, anoint your third eye with this blend and say, *My third eye is open, and I am ready to see the truth.*

Divination Journal

When making divination a regular practice in your life, you'll want to have a journal just for recording your readings, inner visions, and intuitive downloads. This way you can review them all in one place to check the accuracy of your interpretations and fine-tune your intuitive skills.

Journal

3 drops Frankincense

2 drops Sandalwood

2 drops Lavender

1. Select a journal to be your divination journal and mark it as such.
2. Drop the Frankincense, Sandalwood, and Lavender essential oils onto the inside back cover of the journal.
3. Make notes on every reading you do and your interpretations. You can also use this journal to record your dreams, inner journeys, and any intuitive downloads you receive throughout your days. Leave a little space in the margins so you can come back and make notes on how things play out and how your interpretation changes over time, if it does.
4. Periodically revisit your previous readings and make note of any patterns you notice. Each dark moon, refresh the oils on the inside back cover to keep the aroma fresh and potent.

Olfactory Oracle

The oils in this spell are selected to magically enhance your intuition during readings with your tarot or oracle cards. This spell also functions as a blessing or consecration for your deck.

1 drop Helichrysum

1 drop Lavender

1 drop Rosemary

Cotton ball (100 percent cotton)

Deck bag or box

Tarot or oracle deck

1. Drop the Helichrysum, Lavender, and Rosemary essential oils onto the cotton ball, and place the cotton ball in the deck bag with the cards. Say, *May these cards be ever truthful and wise, and may their wisdom shine clearly to my ready, open eyes.*

2. Over time, the cards will absorb the oils so that the aroma will fill the air when they are shuffled and pulled.

3. When you work with the cards, practice relaxing your mind and allowing the inner voice of intuition to speak. Over time, your olfactory memory will help you reach this state more quickly when you work with these scented cards.

Prophetic Dreams Pillow Spray

Spray this on your pillow before you fall asleep to promote vivid, lucid, and prophetic dreams.

15 drops Sandalwood

15 drops Frankincense

10 drops Jasmine

10 drops Lavender

10 drops Helichrysum

1 (2-ounce) glass spray bottle (blue or amber)

2 milliliters polysorbate 20 or 15 milliliters Everclear (emulsifier)

2 ounces distilled water

Amethyst gem chips (optional)

1. Combine the Sandalwood, Frankincense, Jasmine, Lavender, and Helichrysum essential oils in the glass spray bottle and swirl gently to mix.

2. Inhale the synergy and visualize your sleeping body in bed with your third eye wide open, and a beam of sparkling light connecting it and the heavens. Hold the vision and say, *My eyes are closed but still I see, what was and is and what shall be, dreams and visions come to me!*

3. Add the emulsifier, water, and amethyst gem chips (if using). Swirl to mix.

4. Before bed, when you wish to dream, spray your pillow and the air above and repeat the visualization and incantation from step 2. Make sure to write down your experiences in the morning. Even if you don't dream the first few times, writing down your experience will send the signal to your brain that you want to remember your dreams.

Get Intuit Anywhere

Cards, pendulums, tea leaves, dreams . . . they're all great tools for helping us access what our intuitive selves already know. But you don't always have the ability to sit down and perform a full-on reading on every little thing. Sometimes you have to make a decision in the moment, and you need to be able to tell the difference between a gut feeling and the voice of fear. For those moments, there's this very spell.

3 drops Frankincense

1 drop Rosemary

1 drop Black Spruce

Aromatherapy inhaler

1. Add the Frankincense, Rosemary, and Black Spruce essential oils to the wick of an aromatherapy inhaler.
2. Inhale from the wick and relax your mind. On the exhale, say out loud, *I am connected to my highest self, who knows what my soul needs*, or *I trust the signs and synchronicities that appear in my life.*
3. Open your mind to receiving the answer you seek and trust your gut.
4. Whenever you need magical assistance differentiating between the voice of fear and the voice of intuition, pull out this inhaler, take a few deep breaths, and repeat the affirmation (or another intuition affirmation) as needed.

Inner Eye Illumination

Not only are oil-dressed candles good for casting spells, but they're also good for scrying. As your magic candle burns, look to the movement of the flame to garner the answers you seek.

Generally, a strong or growing flame means "yes"; a weak or shrinking flame means "no"; a left-leaning flame indicates answers in the past; a right-leaning flame means more time is needed; flickering means "yes, but with challenges or obstacles"; crackles indicate a spirit present (perhaps reinforcing signs you have already received); a flame leaning away from you is a sign to take action; and a flame leaning toward you means you already know the answer.

Large glass mixing bowl

1 drop Sandalwood

1 drop Helichrysum

1 drop Lavender

1 drop Cedarwood

1 drop Jasmine

¼ teaspoon carrier oil

Beeswax chime candle and holder

Matches or lighter

1. In the large mixing bowl, combine the Sandalwood, Helichrysum, Lavender, Cedarwood, and Jasmine essential oils with the carrier oil and dress the candle (coat it completely with the oil blend).

2. Light the candle someplace where the air is still and let the aroma of the warm oils relax your mind. Focus on your breathing, and on the flame.

3. At this point you can either use some other tool for divination, such as a pendulum or tarot deck, or you can ask a question and divine from the candle itself.

Soothsayer's Soak

This recipe makes five standard-size bath bombs to relax your mind and open your inner eye.

2 large glass mixing bowls

1 cup baking soda

½ cup cornstarch

½ cup Epsom salt

½ cup citric acid

3 tablespoons carrier oil

10 drops Frankincense

10 drops Sandalwood

10 drops Cedarwood

10 drops Lavender

¾ tablespoons water

Bath bomb molds

Moonstone or amethyst crystals (optional)

1. In one large glass mixing bowl, combine the baking soda, cornstarch, Epsom salt, and citric acid.
2. In the second glass mixing bowl, combine the carrier oil, the Frankincense, Sandalwood, Cedarwood, and Lavender essential oils, and the water.
3. Slowly add the dry ingredients to the wet ingredients. While mixing, visualize yourself folding in the sparkling light of divine wisdom. The

mixture should hold its shape when squeezed. Pack tightly into the molds and let set for 1 to 2 minutes before unmolding. Let dry for 24 hours, then store in an airtight container.

4. When you're ready to use each bath bomb, dim the lights and surround yourself with the crystals (if using).

5. Enter the water, submerge the bath bomb, and relax your conscious mind. Visualize the sparkling light from step 3 filling the water and permeating your skin, opening your third eye to receive divine knowledge and wisdom.

6. Lie back, ask a question, and simply allow your open mind to settle on an answer.

Rose Runes

If you love working with runes or have always wanted to learn, you can make your own set with psychic-boosting plant magic! Alternatively, you can carve or stamp other symbols to make an oracle of your choice.

For an in-depth beginner's guide to making, reading, and working with runes, check out my first book, *Modern Runes: Discover the Magic of Casting and Divination for Everyday Life.*

---

2 large glass mixing bowls

1 cup flour

½ cup salt

10 drops Frankincense

10 drops Sandalwood

5 drops Rose

1 tablespoon jojoba oil

¼ to ½ cup water

Carving tool

Cloth pouch or wooden box

---

1. In one glass mixing bowl, combine the flour and salt.
2. In the second mixing bowl, combine the Frankincense, Sandalwood, and Rose essential oils with the jojoba oil.
3. Add the flour mixture to the oil blend and add the water gradually until a clay-like texture is achieved. As you mix, shape, and carve the clay, focus on your intention for this oracle.

4. For an Elder Futhark rune set, form 24 spheres of roughly equal size by rolling chunks of clay between your palms. Then, use your thumb to flatten them into pebble-like discs.

5. With a carving tool such as a small knife or toothpick, carve the shapes of the runes into the discs.

6. Let the discs air-dry for several days, flipping every 24 hours, or dry in a dehydrator at low temperature.

7. Paint or stain the runes themselves but leave most of the clay natural so the oils can breathe. You can mix up another batch of just the oils from this recipe to consecrate and recharge the runes periodically. Between readings, store them in the cloth pouch or wooden box.

SUBSTITUTIONS CHART

BASIL	CLARITY	Eucalyptus, Frankincense, Lemon, Rosemary, Spearmint
	LOVE	Black Pepper, Grapefruit, Orange, Rose, Tangerine
	MONEY	Black Pepper, Frankincense, Grapefruit, Lemon, Orange, Spearmint, Tangerine
BLACK PEPPER	PROTECTION	Cinnamon, Clove, Ginger, Myrrh, Oregano, Peppermint, Tea Tree
	POWER	Cinnamon, Ginger, Peppermint
BLACK SPRUCE	CLEANSING	Spruce (any), Pine, Fir, Juniper, Rosemary, Eucalyptus, Citronella
	INTUITION	Frankincense, Helichrysum, Rosemary, Cedarwood
CARDAMOM	LOVE	Cassia, Ginger, Nutmeg, Orange, Rose
	MONEY	Cassia, Cinnamon, Clove, Ginger, Nutmeg
	HEALING	Ginger, Spearmint, Peppermint
CASSIA	PROTECTION	Black Pepper, Cinnamon, Clove
	LOVE	Cardamom, Nutmeg
	WEALTH	Cinnamon, Clove, Nutmeg
	POWER	Black Pepper, Cardamom, Cinnamon, Clove, Patchouli
CEDARWOOD	SPIRITUALITY	Frankincense, Helichrysum, Myrrh, Sandalwood
	GROUNDING	Frankincense, Vetiver, Patchouli, Myrrh
	HEALING	Lavender, Cedarwood, Davana

CHAMOMILE	WEALTH	Grapefruit, Lemon, Orange, Tangerine, Spearmint
	GOOD VIBES	Bergamot, Cedarwood, Davana, Geranium, Lemon, Orange, Tangerine
CITRONELLA	CLEANSING	Black Spruce, Chamomile, Eucalyptus, Lemon, Lemon Verbena, Lemongrass, Lime, Palmarosa, Peppermint, Tea Tree, Rosemary
CLARY SAGE	MOON MAGIC	Lavender, Jasmine, Rose, Chamomile
	DREAMS & VISIONS	Lavender, Jasmine, Sandalwood, Frankincense, Chamomile
CLOVE	PROTECTION	Black Pepper, Cassia, Cinnamon, Ginger, Patchouli
	LOVE	Cardamom, Cassia, Cinnamon, Ginger, Nutmeg
	WEALTH	Cardamom, Cassia, Cinnamon, Ginger, Nutmeg
EUCALYPTUS	CLEANSING	Black Spruce, Chamomile, Citronella, Lemon, Lemon Verbena, Lemongrass, Peppermint, Tea Tree, Juniper, Fir, Pine, Rosemary
FRANKINCENSE	THIRD EYE	Sandalwood, Helichrysum, Myrrh, Clary Sage, Lavender, Cedarwood
	WEALTH	Myrrh, Cassia
	HEALING	Helichrysum, Lavender, Myrrh
GERANIUM	LOVE	Rose, Ylang Ylang, Neroli, Orange
	FRIENDSHIP	Cistus, Chamomile, Davana, Ylang Ylang, Bergamot, Tangerine, Neroli
	PROTECTION	Chamomile, Rose, Black Pepper, Petitgrain
	GOOD VIBES	Chamomile, Rose, Davana, Ylang Ylang, Bergamot
	LOVE	

GINGER		Cardamom, Cassia, Cinnamon, Nutmeg, Orange
	WEALTH	Cardamom, Cassia, Cinnamon, Clove, Nutmeg
	POWER	Cassia, Cinnamon, Peppermint
HELICHRYSUM	HEALING	Lavender, Myrrh, Frankincense
	INTUITION	Frankincense, Clary Sage, Sandalwood, Lavender, Patchouli
JASMINE	MOON MAGIC	Lavender, Clary Sage, Chamomile
	LOVE	Rose, Ylang Ylang, Neroli, Geranium, Cardamom, Nutmeg
	DREAMS & VISIONS	Lavender, Clary Sage, Sandalwood, Frankincense, Chamomile
LAVENDER	HEALING	Frankincense, Chamomile, Clary Sage, Cedarwood
	INTUITION	Frankincense, Clary Sage, Sandalwood, Cedarwood
LEMON	CLEANSING	Eucalyptus, Lime, Peppermint, Spearmint, Chamomile
	WEALTH	Grapefruit, Orange, Tangerine, Spearmint, Basil, Chamomile, Ginger
MYRRH	PROTECTION	Black Pepper, Cassia, Cinnamon, Clove, Patchouli
	HEALING	Frankincense, Lavender, Helichrysum
NUTMEG	LOVE	Cardamom, Cassia, Ginger, Jasmine, Patchouli, Vanilla, Rose
	WEALTH	Cardamom, Cassia, Cinnamon, Clove, Ginger
ORANGE	LOVE	Tangerine, Geranium, Rose, Neroli, Jasmine, Cardamom, Basil, Ginger
	WEALTH	Tangerine, Basil, Ginger, Cardamom, Clove
	GOOD VIBES	Tangerine, Bergamot, Lemon, Lime, Grapefruit

PATCHOULI	GROUNDING	Cedarwood, Frankincense, Vetiver, Myrrh
	WEALTH	Frankincense, Myrrh, Vetiver, Ginger, Cardamom, Cassia, Cinnamon
	LOVE	Nutmeg, Jasmine, Rose, Vanilla, Cardamom, Ginger, Cassia
PEPPERMINT	CLEANSING	Black Spruce, Chamomile, Citronella, Eucalyptus, Lemon, Lemon Verbena, Lemongrass, Tea Tree, Juniper, Fir, Pine, Rosemary
	POWER	Black Pepper, Cassia, Cinnamon, Ginger
	WEALTH	Basil, Spearmint, Ginger, Orange
ROSE	LOVE	Geranium, Ylang Ylang, Neroli, Jasmine, Palmarosa
	PROTECTION	Geranium, Palmarosa, Black Pepper, Myrrh
ROSEMARY	CLEANSING	Black Spruce, Chamomile, Citronella, Eucalyptus, Lemon Verbena, Lemongrass, Tea Tree, Lavender, Juniper, Fir, Pine, Peppermint
	CLARITY	Basil, Eucalyptus, Frankincense, Lemon, Spearmint
SAGE	WISDOM	Cedarwood, Clary Sage, Frankincense, Rosemary
	BLESSING	Cedarwood, Frankincense, Palo Santo, Sandalwood
SANDALWOOD	INTUITION	Frankincense, Lavender, Clary Sage
	BLESSING	Cedarwood, Frankincense, Palo Santo, Sage
SPEARMINT	CLEANSING	Peppermint, Spruce, Juniper, Pine, Fir, Eucalyptus, Citronella, Lemongrass
	WEALTH	Basil, Ginger, Orange, Peppermint
VETIVER	GROUNDING	Cedarwood, Frankincense, Myrrh, Patchouli
	WEALTH	Frankincense, Myrrh, Ginger, Cardamom, Patchouli

YLANG YLANG	LOVE	Geranium, Rose, Neroli, Jasmine

GLOSSARY

carrier oil: This type of oil is any of several plant-derived fatty oils used to dilute EOs for topical or internal use.

emulsifier: A compound that enables oil and water to mix without separating. An emulsifier is necessary to make water-based sprays with EOs.

EO: This abbreviation stands for essential oil.

EVOO: This abbreviation stands for extra-virgin olive oil, which is used as a carrier oil.

FCO: This abbreviation stands for fractionated coconut oil (coconut oil in liquid form), which is used as a carrier oil.

hot oil: Any essential oils that are known to create a sensation of heat or cold on the skin or are known to frequently cause skin irritation when not properly diluted are considered hot oils.

neat: This describes the method of applying undiluted essential oils.

olfactory memory: This type of memory is the persistent and highly intuitive recollection of odors and associated experiences.

phototoxicity: This quality describes items that cause increased light absorption, sometimes resulting in burns or discoloration.

qi: This is the subtle energy found in all things, living and nonliving. Some things have very strong positive qi, some things have strong negative qi, and some things have weaker qi, which can lean either way.

sensitization: This is the process by which some people, over time and extended usage, develop a sensitivity to an oil they have used many times before without issue.

synergy: This is when a blend of EOs has been allowed to mix and harmonize for some time (from a few minutes to a few days) without the addition of a carrier oil. Carrier oils can be added to blended synergies for topical use, or a blended synergy can be diffused or applied for certain purposes as is.

RESOURCES

Oil Coven

VervainAndTheRoses.com/oilcoven

Oil Coven is a space for witches to learn and grow together, harnessing plant magic and the power of community to manifest a more beautiful and magical future for all. We gather mostly online, and members have access to a wide variety of exclusive events and resources for plant magic and oil education, including classes, giveaways, and moon circles, plus membership pricing on some of the best oils around.

The Essential Oil Truth: The Facts Without the Hype by Jen O'Sullivan

Everything you've ever wanted to know about essential oil sourcing, usage, distillation, quality, and more, presented in 48 easy-to-understand mini-lessons.

French Aromatherapy: Essential Oil Recipes & Usage Guide by Jen O'Sullivan

A helpful guide for learning to incorporate essential oils into your daily life for personal health and wellness, including internal and external use.

The School for Aromatic Studies

AromaticStudies.com

Founded by aromatherapist Jade Shutes and certified by the NAHA (National Association for Holistic Aromatherapy), this school offers a free online introduction to aromatherapy and multiple options for those interested in deeper learning or certification.

Blackthorn's Botanical Magic: The Green Witch's Guide to Essential Oils for Spellcraft, Ritual & Healing by Amy Blackthorn

Of the many titles on this subject, I recommend this one for the aspiring oil witch. The oil profiles especially are rich in lore and suggestions for magical use.

The Oily Crystal: Safe Blending of Essential Oils and Crystals for People and Pets by Allie Phillips
This 32-page booklet is worth hunting down if you care to devise your own spells combining crystals and essential oils, as it details the safety information you will need to know to safely combine the two for internal and external use.

Llewellyn's Complete Book of Correspondences: A Comprehensive & Cross-Referenced Resource for Pagans & Wiccans by Sandra Kynes
A reference book of magical correspondences is invaluable for creating your own spells. From colors to creatures and planets to plants, this book is designed to help you select spell elements that correspond to your intention.

The Complete List of Essential Oil Substitutes
SacredSoulHolistics.co.uk/blogs/news/essential-oil-substitutes
This web page offers substitutions for more than 80 essential oils based on intended usage. Its focus is aromatherapeutic rather than magical, but as aromatherapeutic effects often complement magical effects, you may find it useful. I certainly have!

Modern Runes: Discover the Magic of Casting and Divination for Everyday Life by Vervain Helsdottir
One of my favorite oil magic practices is to apply oils from enchanted roller bottles to my skin in the shapes of runes appropriate for my intention. If you want to experiment with this practice or learn to use your Rose Runes, this book will start you down the path.

REFERENCES

Filiptsova, O. V., L. V. Gazzavi-Rogozina, I. A. Timoshyna, O. I. Naboka, Ye. V. Dyomina, and A. V. Ochkur. "The Essential Oil of Rosemary and Its Effect on the Human Image and Numerical Short-Term Memory." *Egyptian Journal of Basic and Applied Sciences* 4, no. 2 (2017): 107–111. doi.org/10.1016/j.ejbas.2017.04.002.

O'Sullivan, Jen. *The Essential Oil Truth: The Facts without the Hype.* 31 Oils, LLC, 2018.

Tisserand, Robert, and Rodney Young. *Essential Oil Safety: A Guide for Health Care Professionals.* Edinburgh, UK: Churchill Livingstone, Elsevier, 2014.